WHY
POSTNATAL
RECOVERY
MATTERS

Sophie Messager

pinter
&
martin

Why Postnatal Recovery Matters (Pinter & Martin Why It Matters 18)

First published by Pinter & Martin Ltd 2020

©2020 Sophie Messager

ISBN 978-1-78066-625-9

Also available as an ebook

Pinter & Martin Why It Matters ISSN 2056-8657
Series editor: Susan Last
Index: Helen Bilton
Cover Design: Blok Graphic, London
Cover illustration: Lucy Davey
Author photograph: Ali Dover www.alidover.com

British Library Cataloguing-in-Publication Data

A catalogue record for this book is available from the British Library.

Set in Minion

Printed and bound in the EU by Hussar

This book has been printed on paper that is sourced and harvested from sustainable forests and is FSC accredited.

Pinter & Martin Ltd
6 Effra Parade
London SW2 1PS

pinterandmartin.com

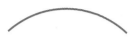

Contents

Birth produces two people. The first: a flailing soul, struggling to take in a new world, a new way of being. The second: a baby. Bunmi Laditan

Birth is about so much more than the wriggling of a tiny body out of a larger one. When we birth, we don't just birth babies. We birth ourselves, we birth our families and we reshape our lives. Dr Sara Wickham

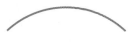

Introduction

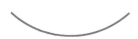

A tale of two births

A baby is born. While the new mother was pregnant, she was the centre of attention. Now she is elbowed out of the way by visitors who just want to hold her baby. Visitors mean she misses out on naps, and they expect her to entertain them, leaving her with a messy house and a cranky baby. Nobody asks her how she feels. With no previous experience of babies, and no family nearby, she feels lost and worries whether she is doing things right. Her partner returns to work after two short weeks. She struggles to meet her baby's needs, and her own. Nobody helps with the chores or the cooking. She receives a lot of gifts, but they are all for the baby. She is exhausted by the broken nights, and longs for a much-needed nap, or some baby-free time. Her days are a blur of feeding and baby care. Her social network has disappeared, as her friends are all working 9 to 5 jobs. She feels isolated and lonely. She longs for adult company. She feels guilty that she isn't enjoying every moment. She struggles to make sense of this new experience. She hides her feelings and pretends everything is okay. Everybody gives her conflicting advice and undermines her instincts. Nobody takes care of her body, and there is immense pressure to 'go back to normal' both physically and socially. By the time a month has passed, she is exhausted, uncertain about her mothering skills and still in a fresh postpartum state physically and emotionally.

Postnatal care is the poor relation of the birth world. Our culture focuses entirely on the baby rather than the needs of the new mother. This is reflected very strongly in the fact that the majority of the gifts given to new parents are baby clothes and toys. Yet babies do not care for plush toys and clothing: what they need most, beyond warmth, shelter and food, are loving carers. In order to be able to nurture their babies, parents themselves need to be supported, nurtured, and cared for. Surely attention and gifts, rather than being directed at the baby, ought to be directed at the parents, and most importantly at the mother? This wisdom is still part of many cultures around the world. It used to be part of Western culture too, but it has been lost in favour of a culture which glorifies a mother who 'gets back to normal' as soon as possible after birth as if nothing had happened. This book is an argument for a change to a more supportive, nurturing postpartum culture.

A baby is born. The new mother is celebrated and her status is enhanced by motherhood. There is an understanding that she has performed an incredible feat by growing and birthing a whole new person, and that she needs time, rest and good care and nutrition to recover well. Family members, and members of her community, rally round. Everything in her house is taken care of: all the chores and all the cooking. All she has to do is rest and get to know her baby. Experienced mothers surround her and support her in learning to care for and feed her baby. Someone comes daily to massage her body, and bind her abdomen with a cloth, in ways designed to help her recover faster, both physically and spiritually. She is treated and revered like a queen. People fight over who is cooking her next meal. The dishes are specifically designed to restore her strength, nourish her body and boost her health. She is never alone: there is always adult company, and she can talk about her feelings and make sense of her changing sense of self. There are loving arms to hold the baby whenever she needs it. She recovers well, and by the time a month has passed, and she is ready to re-enter community life, she is stronger, confident and competent at caring for her baby.

This comparison may sound too polarised, or too idealistic, but I cobbled together the stories from years of listening to mothers from many different cultures. I remember chatting to a lovely woman from Kenya in the school playground. She told me a harrowing tale of the contrast between her experiences after giving birth to her first child in Kenya, and having her second in the UK. She told me that people fought over who would cook you dinner, and she said you didn't even have to wash yourself. When she moved to the UK and her second child was born, she had no family nearby. She had an older child to take to preschool, and a husband who expected a hot dinner on the table every night. She felt utterly lonely, desperately missed the community and the postnatal support back home, and cried every day.

Over the last 10 years I have supported many women on their journey to motherhood and I have listened to hundreds of stories. I have witnessed the same struggle to adjust, and the same guilt at 'not doing anything productive'. I have seen and heard women feeling and saying the exact things I felt myself as a new mother.

I was incredibly gifted after the birth of my second baby because my mother-in-law from India was here. She told me to go to bed with my baby and stay there. She never let me cook. She did everything including holding the baby. She advised me to wrap my belly. Keep warm. And to not allow visitors to hold baby and pass her around. My husband made me super food balls. I had placenta smoothie and encapsulation and 'closing the bones'. Seema Barua

I had all the support I could have asked for, and I had a wonderful easing into motherhood. Deborah Neiger

I had a wonderful independent midwife who told me to stay in bed for a week after my birth ('As soon as they see you dressed and downstairs your postnatal recovery will be over', she told me.) She said to leave a key under the mat with a note saying 'Make tea on your way up, stay no longer than 30 mins.' It was going really well until an old friend's husband said 'Why are you in bed still? Are you ill? You've only had a baby, which is physiological, so you don't need to stay in bed'. This misogynist comment made me feel so shitty and pathetic – unworthy of rest. Sophia MacDonnell

I was deeply upset that nobody could see the hurt and pain I was in. From friends and family to health

professionals – they missed the emotional and physical pain I was experiencing and how overwhelmed I was. And that made me feel really selfish – how could I resent a baby because nobody was looking after me?! Our society isn't set up to look after new moms, especially first timers. Meg Hill

I remember when my husband went back to work. Sometimes he would ask what we'd been up to (it might be around 11am). He would ask me if we were even dressed yet. I used to feel so bad saying no (even though he never did anything to make me feel bad), that I would get my son and I dressed with the 5am feed, and then we would both go back to bed dressed for the day. It felt more acceptable to say we had a little snooze mid-morning than to say we hadn't really started the day. Nicola Witcombe

It took me at least one and a half years to recover as it was a caesarean section. There was no effective support from the healthcare services: they could not even recognise that our baby was starving. We were living alone here in the UK without any kind of family background. My pure luck was that we had a friend who acted as a private midwife and my husband is a medical doctor still fixing me with Chinese medicine. Ilona Vero

When I started working as a doula, I was struck by how many women struggle in silence, because they think they are the only ones who are finding things difficult, and feel ashamed of it.

I was once doula to an American woman called Emma. She was a fun, intelligent woman, with a wicked sense of humour. During one of my postnatal visits, when her daughter was three months old and her son was three years old, as we were trying to chat while she was feeding her daughter and entertaining her son with puzzles, Emma told me that she didn't understand why she was so tired all the time. I said 'You're tired because you have a three-month-old and a three-year-old!'. She replied, 'But everybody else seems to be coping better than me'. I explained that this wasn't true, and that everybody else was lying, or pretending. Emma also told me that she felt guilty asking for support.

I believe that our culture, with its insidious 'picture perfect' social media images, creates a system which perpetuates the myth of perfect motherhood. Nobody shares the bad moments, so it's easy to think that everyone else is having an easier time than you, feel shame that you aren't coping and hide these feelings, which leads to a vicious cycle of falseness and feelings of inadequacy.

The more I worked supporting new mothers, the more incensed I became about the lack of support and their silent struggle. Because I'm very curious by nature, I started asking every foreign mother I met about her culture's traditions of postpartum recovery. The stories I heard left me flabbergasted. Swati told me that when her twins were born in India, her mum hired an old lady from the village to come and give her a full body massage every day for a month! I tell this story to expectant parents because it really illustrates what we are missing out on.

I am married to Chi, who was born in Hong Kong, and I have supported a handful of Chinese clients as a doula. The Chinese tradition of *zuò yuè zi* (Mandarin) or *co jyut zi* (Cantonese), which translates as 'doing the month' is a complex mix of rest, binding, very specific nutritious food and keeping the mother warm.

The more stories I heard, the more strongly I felt that our culture was letting new mothers down. Most of us have no idea that the support we are receiving is not adequate. We don't realise that we aren't getting what we need. We are grateful for the flowers, babygros or stuffed toys, without understanding that home-cooked food and help with the washing up would be better.

Anna was a new mum. Her baby daughter was a couple of weeks old. She had gone for a much-needed nap. Her baby was asleep in a sling on my chest. I had done some tidying up and I was keen to make her something warming and hearty for lunch, perhaps soup. I opened her fridge and it was nearly empty. When she woke up, I pointed at the many bouquets of flowers in her kitchen, and said 'those sure are pretty, but you can't eat them'. Every time I visited, she asked me to throw wilted flowers away. The bouquets seemed to me to be a symbol of the misplaced focus of the 'support' new mothers were receiving.

I became determined to change things. I wrote blogs, I posted on social media. I tried to raise awareness. But it wasn't enough. This book was born from the desire to reach more people, especially new and expectant parents, in the hope that we can start to change the way we support postpartum women in our culture.

I share stories and quotes from women from the UK, but also from cultures where truly nurturing postpartum care still exists, in the hope that it may inspire women to ask for this kind of support, and encourage those around them to offer it. I have a scientific background, and I am fascinated by how scientific evidence and traditional knowledge overlap. This book therefore contains many references to papers and books about postpartum recovery. However, some of the practices advocated by tradition do not (yet) have any research to back them up. Nevertheless, similar practices often exist around the world, which suggests that there is real knowledge and wisdom behind them. Just because something hasn't been studied, doesn't mean that it isn't effective. Follow your instincts on what feels right for your mind and body.

I am acutely aware that most of us do not live in close-knit communities, and that many of us live away from our families. Therefore the 'ideal picture' I describe above is probably impossible to recreate in its entirety. However, I firmly believe that is possible to benefit from even small changes to postnatal care, and I aim to demonstrate that the way to have a restorative postpartum period boils down to taking care of four simple aspects: rest, nutrition, social support and bodywork. These chapters are the core of the book. I have tried to arrange a buffet of options for you to pick and choose from to suit your own circumstances, focusing mainly on the first four to six weeks after birth, although I recognise that full postpartum recovery lasts a lot longer. One great way to help ensure that you get the kind of support you need and want is to write a postnatal recovery plan, and in the chapter about this I give lots of ideas and examples to help you.

If you are reading this book as an expectant or new parent, I hope that it will help you think ahead about some of the things you can put in place so that you have an easier, more supported experience after your baby is born.

If you are a friend, or a family member of an expectant or new mother, I hope that this book will help you think about ways that you can offer support after the birth.

If you are a birth worker, doula, midwife, health professional, educator, antenatal or postnatal course facilitator or therapist, or anybody who works with and supports families, I hope that this book will provide a framework for you to encourage your clients to think and plan for the postnatal period, and that it will add useful ideas to your practice.

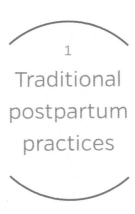

1
Traditional postpartum practices

'Because you and your baby are emotionally and physically vulnerable, you will be wise to follow certain guidelines. No matter where or how you had your baby, a long period of postpartum nurturing is essential' Robin Lim

'Ritual is a very important part of culture, and the rituals of social transition are present in every society. They relate to changes in the life cycle and in social position, thus linking the physiological and social aspects of an individual's life. Childbirth signals a major life cycle transition for a woman, irrespective of the culture to which she belongs' (Huang, 2010)

Once upon a time, all around the world, new mothers were celebrated and nurtured. Yes, even in the Western world. Nowadays there seems to be a misguided belief that these practices are 'exotic' and outdated, and found only in developing world cultures. However, the fact that traditional postpartum practices are common to every continent should give us pause for thought.

Cambridge, where I live, is a very multicultural city, and I have had the opportunity to talk to many mothers about their experiences. I am fascinated by the similarities between traditional practices across the world. The ingredients used to cook a postpartum dish might be different, but the aim is always to replenish the new mother. Different methods and cloths are using for binding, but binding is universal. Different people come to support the new mother, but there is an underlying wisdom that rest is paramount, and other people should take care of household chores. There is also an understanding that social support is essential and the new mother cannot manage alone.

In many cultures, there is an acknowledgement that the weeks after birth represent a unique window during which, if properly cared for, a woman has a chance to replenish herself – to reset – with long-term consequences for her health and wellbeing.

Published research agrees with these observations. The abstract for a review paper about traditional postpartum practices and rituals (Dennis et al, 2007) states that:

Many cultures around the world observe specific postpartum rituals to avoid ill health in later years. This qualitative systematic review examined the literature describing traditional postpartum practices from 51 studies in over 20 different countries. Commonalities were identified in practices across cultures. Specifically, the themes included organized support for the mother, periods of rest, prescribed food to be eaten or prohibited, hygiene practices and those related to infant care and breastfeeding, among others. These rituals allow the mother to be 'mothered' for a period of time after the birth. They may have beneficial health effects as well as facilitate the transition to motherhood. In today's society, with modernization, migration and globalization, individuals may be unable to carry out the rituals or, conversely, feel pressured to carry out activities in which they no longer believe. The understanding of traditional postpartum practices can inform the provision of culturally competent perinatal services.

Interestingly, the authors of published literature on traditional postpartum practices are often quick to dismiss those traditional practices. Our culture tends to embrace all things scientific as 'truth', and dismiss anything not studied by modern science as worthless.

In an article about 'doing the month' in China (Guodong Ding et al, 2018) the authors write:

Although many of the practices and rituals of doing the month have been disproved by science or common sense, many Chinese follow the ancestral rituals because they are part of their culture and traditional principles that guide everyday life.

As a scientist I find this irritating, because there is very little research on the effects of following a traditional postpartum month as a whole (apart from some limited research on the effect on mental health). This isn't a scientific way to look at things. Lack of published evidence isn't the same thing as proof of lack of effectiveness. And many other publications show protective effects of traditional postpartum practices on physical and mental wellbeing (Raven, 2007; Grigoriadis et al, 2009).

Anthropologist Eleanor Fleming introduced me to the

WEIRD societies acronym, which was coined by anthropologist Joseph Henrich in a paper called 'The weirdest people in the world?' (Henrich and Heine, 2010). It stands for Western, Educated, Industrialised, Rich, and Democratic. In the review, the authors found that 96 percent of subjects in behavioural science research were from Western industrialised countries. Yet these countries only represent 12 percent of the world's population! So we must be careful about the conclusions we draw when trying to study 'normal' human behaviour.

Cultures that understand that new mothers need a special kind of support also recognise that the mother herself undergoes a tremendous transformation, akin to a metamorphosis, when she gives birth. As a doula I've sometimes explained to parents that becoming a mother is a bit like being a teenager. You're stuck between two states and have lost your sense of identity, and it can feel uncomfortable at times. In the birth world some people refer to becoming a mother as a 'caterpillar to butterfly' process; I personally prefer the phoenix analogy. In her book *Broken Open: how difficult times can help us grow*, Elizabeth Lesser describes the experience like this:

> *I call it the Phoenix Process – in honor of the mythic bird with golden plumage whose story has been told throughout the ages. The Egyptians called the bird the Phoenix, and believed that every 500 years the Phoenix bird renewed his quest for his true self. Knowing that a new way could only be found with the death of his worn-out habits, defenses, and beliefs, the Phoenix built a pyre of cinnamon and myrrh, sat in the flames, and burned to death. Then he rose from the ashes as a new being – a strange amalgam of who he had been before, and who he had become. A new bird, yet ever more himself; changed, and at the same time, the eternal Phoenix.*

I like this for two reasons: first, because the new phoenix will probably look exactly the same to the untrained eye, unlike the butterfly and the caterpillar. New mothers may also look the same to the outside world, with the tremendous change inside largely invisible. Second, when I picture the newborn phoenix, I see a small, chick-like bird, tentative and flailing. This evokes more of a 'need to nurture' than a full-grown butterfly.

Traditional postpartum support usually lasts between 30 and 40 days, and can be categorised into four main areas: rest, food, bodywork, and social support. These categories overlap. For instance, when it comes to rest and social support, having relatives (usually women) coming to help during the postpartum period means that there is another pair of hands to cook, do chores, hold the baby or entertain older children while the new mother rests. It also means that the mother is never alone. Being alone with a new baby and trying to meet the intense needs of a newborn, while recovering from pregnancy and birth and trying to look after yourself, is a near-impossible task.

The 'rest' aspect comes from the understanding that a new mother is recovering from growing and birthing a baby, which takes time, just as it would for someone who had undertaken an enormous physical feat. It also acknowledges the fact that her sleep is being disrupted by caring for her new baby and that she needs more sleep during the day.

When it comes to food and nutrition, growing and birthing a baby can deplete the mother of essential nutrients, and she may well lose some blood during the birth. Traditional postpartum foods are designed to be nourishing, and are similar to foods given to any convalescent or recovering person, being nutrient dense, warm and rich in iron. The food is also designed to support the onset of breastfeeding.

The emphasis on bodywork acknowledges the tremendous

changes a mother's body has gone through to grow and birth a baby, and then to reverse those changes once the baby is born. There are traditional massages, akin to empirical osteopathy, as well as binding practices, found on every continent. We used to have this in the West too, but it has been forgotten. There is also an understanding that the mother has lost of a lot of 'heat' after giving birth, so keeping her warm is paramount.

The social support aspect recognises that being alone isn't normal, and that, as well as needing support around the house so they can rest, new mothers are learning to mother and care for their babies and need other experienced mothers around them.

In her book *The Golden Month*, author Jenny Allison interviews a mother from Mali:

I had ten children, and never had any problems. My mother-in-law looked after me very well and whenever I gave birth, she helped me. She usually massaged me daily as long as I needed for the first 40 days. She fed me chicken soup, fish soup, and eggs. With this complete care, I gave birth ten times without any problems. For 40 days, all I would do was feed my baby and lie next to him or her. I did nothing, no work at all, not even domestic work.

Chinese culture still has a strong tradition of postpartum support, called 'doing the month', which incorporates all four strands. There is a lot of focus on food in particular. The emphasis on keeping warm is strong too, with women being warned against taking baths or drinking cold drinks. Warming foods (such as ginger and ginseng) are given. My mother-in-law told me about warm oil massages and showed me how she wrapped her abdomen with a towel, and when I visited Hong

Kong a couple of years ago I found that a type of Indonesian abdominal massage called Jamu was available in packages of between five and 20 visits for new mothers, and the therapist would visit the new mother's home. Traditionally, a mother's own mother, or mother-in-law, would actually move in to support a new mother, but today it's also common to hire a woman for support (much like a postnatal doula), or to move into one of the postpartum hotels.

I supported Annabel, a new mother from China, as a doula. Annabel had wanted a Chinese doula, but there wasn't one in Cambridge and I was the next best thing being married to a Chinese man. Annabel was keen to follow the tradition as closely as possible. She even cut her hair short in preparation (long hair and not taking showers don't mix!). She prepared some of the main dishes herself in advance, including pig's trotters in black vinegar (a dish rich in nutrients and collagen). Annabel's baby was born by caesarean after a long labour, and complications meant that she had to stay in hospital for a week. I visited every day, carrying her baby in a sling around the ward so that her husband could have a lunch break and Annabel could have a nap. I brought takeaway boxes of traditional Chinese dishes that I had prepared at home so she didn't have to eat the hospital food. I ended up supporting Annabel for several months, and I was amazed by the large parcels of food her family sent her to make sure that she could observe the tradition.

In this book I refer to other cultures only as examples and don't consider them in detail: there are other books that look at this in depth, and you can find references in the further reading section at the end of the book. Instead I look more closely at the four main areas of postpartum recovery. One reason for this is that I do not believe that following a particular 'recipe' from one culture is helpful unless it appeals to you personally. Working with new mothers has taught me that we are all different, and prescriptive advice can be disempowering. Therefore my aim is to give you an overview, like a buffet laid out in front of you, and if a particular approach appeals to you, you can delve deeper into it by reading more elsewhere.

While I believe there is much to be gained from reclaiming traditional postpartum practices, I do not want to paint a picture of 'the old ways' being perfect. Many new mothers feel anxious about their ability to parent, and struggle to adapt to the huge change in their sense of self and identity that comes with motherhood. In this context, being pressured to carry out activities that do not suit them may be a source of stress. For example, some postpartum practices include secluding the mother in her home for a month. While that might be lovely for some, other mothers might find it very hard and experience 'cabin fever' and restlessness.

One of my favourite books about postnatal recovery, *The First Forty Days*, is by Chinese-American author Heng Ou. While it leans heavily towards the traditional Chinese postpartum approach, it incorporates other approaches and recipes. Ou has this to say:

The way forward will not involve mothers-in-law or aunties moving in with their cooking pots. (...) The pattern of the dutiful daughter (or daughter-in-law) and older matriarchs ruling the roost has changed, and while the elders' wisdom can help us find the way, we are in the driver's seat now. Women today are responsible for a complex web of demands, and surrendering to someone else's law for six weeks simply doesn't fit the reality of our lives. (...) Importantly it has to fold in a sixth insight: intuition. It must be orientated to helping the mother tap into her own needs.

Lorraine, a new mother from Singapore, told me stories of women becoming depressed while being forced to undergo the stricter aspects of Chinese confinement:

I refused the traditional Chinese postpartum because it was very restrictive. Some of the confinement nannies – perhaps to be useful, would hand the baby over to the mother (in the middle of the night) only after sussing out if baby is dirty/too hot/too cold etc, by which time the baby is already in an almost inconsolable state. The confinement nanny also washes the baby etc., things I feel that are bonding. When the month is nearly up, most new mothers panic because they feel like they are not ready and haven't been prepared just because they haven't been doing babycare for the past month.

As a doula, I have always understood that each family's needs are different. So I offer things and intuitively gauge whether it is something the mother might like. If the vibe I get is that it is not, I do not push or offer it again. Sadly, I have witnessed well-meaning family members and health professionals giving blanket advice to new mothers, which I know they mean to be helpful, but which may not suit a particular mother.

I once supported a woman called Lydia. Originally from Germany, she was intelligent and articulate and knew what was right for her. She was very good at finding and analysing evidence-based babycare suggestions. We had enjoyable conversations about research, but also about more traditional herbal remedies from Germany. Lydia's experience of new motherhood was made more challenging by the fact that her partner worked away all week. She was a quiet woman who liked her own company, and I wasn't concerned about her mental health because she seemed happy, and had found a creative way of managing her time with her daughter that worked well for both of them. I was at her house when her baby was a few weeks old, when a health professional came to visit and told her she needed to go out more, perhaps to 'have a coffee in Waitrose'. I remember being bemused by this, because it didn't feel like something Lydia would enjoy. Afterwards I asked 'Is having a coffee in Waitrose something you'd like to do?', and she said no. This experience stayed with me, because it exemplifies how hard it is to provide true support when you do not know the person. Well-meaning advice can be very wide of the mark.

> *I found the constant questions of 'are you getting out to any baby groups?' both frustrating and unhelpful. Firstly, I'm trying to figure out life with a new baby, learning to feed them etc – getting out the house is hard enough, let alone for a specific time. Secondly, I didn't particularly want to sit and make idle chit chat with women I don't know about the colour of babies' poo, while pretending my newborn is aware of the 'Wheels on the Bus' that's playing when I hadn't showered in three days, had no sleep and just wanted to sit on the sofa.* India Reynolds

So what I've tried to do is to distil the essence of what is good about traditional postpartum wisdom, while making sure the practices used are nurturing and empowering for anyone who wants to try them. I encourage you to pick and choose to make a unique 'patchwork quilt' of support that will support your transition to motherhood.

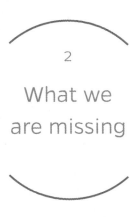

2

What we
are missing

The moment a child is born, the mother is also born. She never existed before. The woman existed, but the mother, never. A mother is something absolutely new. Osho

Care of mothers after childbirth is an issue of universal social importance. Good care in the six-week postpartum period is crucial to the mother's health and wellbeing, and can have lasting benefits, not only for her health, and relationship with her newborn baby, but more widely, for her family and community as well. Jenny Allison

Once upon a time in the UK we had the same postpartum system in place as I described in the previous chapter. A period of at least a month after the birth, during which the family/community rallied around so all we had to do was rest, safe in the knowledge that another pair of hands was available to hold the baby, be fed nutritious replenishing foods, get to know our new baby and, supported by experienced women, build confidence in our new role as a mother. As little as a hundred years ago there was a tradition known as 'lying in', which lasted between two weeks and two months.

For example, in Scotland in the second half of the 18th century and the first half of the 19th century:

It was customary for the new mother to lie-in for a month after the delivery. Owing to the popular perception that the act of childbirth rendered her 'unclean', she could neither share the marital bed during this period nor perform her usual household tasks, which were therefore carried out by her husband, her friends, or perhaps by a paid nurse. In England, as Wilson points out, she was generally confined to bed in the warm, darkened birthing chamber for between three and fourteen days, during which time only female visitors were permitted. (...) Her month of seclusion culminated with her 'churching', after which ceremony she was fully re-integrated into society. (Cameron, 2003)

Warmth, interestingly, was also considered important in the West. Midwife Siobhan Taylor told me:

The importance of keeping warm after birth is something that was still considered important in California 25 years ago. On the delivery ward where I worked they had a 6 feet high warming oven where they put flannelette sheets. These were used to wrap the mum in once she had given birth. It helped with the shivery/shaky stage that so many women experience and helped the body to birth the placenta.

In Europe and America, there was historically a tradition of communal and neighbourly reciprocal support during pregnancy and the postpartum, which lasted into the 19th century. The rise of urbanisation and class stratification started the trend for hired help rather than community support. By the 20th century, social support had mostly gone. In colonial America, the lying-in period lasted six to eight weeks, during which the woman rested and other members of the community took care of the household and other children (Placksin, 1998).

In the UK there are vestiges of the 40-day 'lying-in' period. In 1902, UK legislation on midwifery practice defined ten days as the necessary time for lying in after the birth, during which period the mother was expected to rest and to receive attention from a midwife. It seems that women highly valued this time (Marks, 1996), but developments in maternity care and the routines of hospital practice have resulted in other arrangements, such as 24-hour transfer home from hospital. Many women in the UK now resume household duties by the end of the first week after giving birth, and few have the benefit of support from female relatives living nearby. They do not generally receive as much care from their mothers by comparison with the traditional arrangements for Chinese mothers (Huang and Mathers, 2010).

In the UK, we used to have monthly nurses, who were hired for a month after the birth to look after the new mother. Genealogist and historian Elizabeth Walne explains:

I was intrigued by the concept of the monthly nurse, as in as little as three generations, the term has pretty much fallen out of use. Those that I have spoken to have not had a clue about the duties of these women, perhaps surprising as only a century ago there were over 5,000 monthly nurses in London alone. (…) I looked at numbers in 1901. A staggering 22,300 were recorded as monthly nurses on the schedule this time around (...). Only a year later, changes to the status of midwifery began the process of transforming the care of women and babies which eventually saw the occupation drop off the radar and the arrival of our modern care processes. (Walne, 2011)

Midwife Becky Reed interviewed her own mother, who gave birth near Cambridge in 1951. Her mother explained that 'one thing that was very different is that you were expected to remain bedridden for about a fortnight – and really bedridden, you weren't expected to do anything much at all'. Her mother went on to say that they had a lady provided by the council (but they had to pay for her) known as a visiting home help, who came to look after her and the house during that time.

Becky herself gave birth in 1976, when the norm was to stay in hospital for ten days after the birth. Her mother then came to look after her at home. Becky also mentioned that in the 1980s in the UK, midwives visited new mothers at home twice a day for the first week, and then daily until ten days.

Midwife Siobhan Taylor tells a similar story. When her granny gave birth in the 1940s, she had a lying-in period of two weeks and a maternity nurse was hired to look after her.

As the length of stay in hospital after birth has steadily reduced, it hasn't been replaced by care in the home. Surveys show that women are critical of the postnatal care they receive compared to birth care. The impact of the reduction in the length of time women spend in hospital doesn't appear to have been studied adequately (Byrom et al, 2010).

Today, not only does our culture not offer any practical support to new mothers, but it also puts immense pressure on them to 'get on with it', which can lead to feelings of guilt, shame and inadequacy. Worse, people who are struggling tend to not admit to it, as it is perceived as a sign of weakness.

If you are reading this as a new mother, and you are struggling, I would like you to know this: there is nothing wrong with you, this isn't your fault. Our society as a whole isn't working to support new families properly. This isn't a criticism of the health system, because I know that midwives and health visitors go above and beyond to support women as best as they can in an underfunded and understaffed system. It is our society that needs to wake up and understand the need for more holistic support for new mothers.

As a culture, the focus of our support is wrong. While pregnant a woman's growing belly may be the centre of attention, but once the baby has been born the focus shifts almost entirely to the baby. There is no acknowledgement that the mother is new and fragile too, and needs the same care and attention as her baby.

When I was working in Home Based Childcare as a Visiting Teacher, I once asked a new mum what the most beneficial things about my visits had been. Her answer broke my heart. 'I knew you were coming to see how the nanny was getting on (this family had twins and a one-year-old so qualified for some free nanny hours), but I pretended you were my friend coming to visit. One day you bought me a magazine and I wept, because of your kindness. You visited every month, just getting a visitor was the highlight of the month. The day I cried when you asked how I was, was the day I realized I needed help; no one else looked at me and asked how I was'. Mums of multiples are often overwhelmed with isolation, expectations and exhaustion. Everyone looks at the babies, but few see the mamas. Bronwyn Wills-Tiddy

This is very obvious when you look at the presents given to new families: baby cards, stuffed toys, baby clothes, bouquets of flowers. None of these nurture the mother. The same is true of 'baby showers' organised during pregnancy. Visitors are often keen to cuddle the new baby, but few ask the mother how she feels and what she needs. Not many will check whether she needs a nap or a shower, or think about bringing food, or offer to do a load of laundry, wash some dishes or take out the rubbish. Many expect to be entertained and offered refreshments.

> *I remember so vividly after the birth of my first son how my sister came over and did not ask me once how I was. She picked him up, took a million photos for Instagram and bought him a toy. For a whole year I never heard the words 'How are you?'. I even made her tea for her at three days postpartum.* Azeeta Nielsen

> *I remember when my son was a month old a lot of relatives asking when I was going back to work and them always commenting on my weight like I wasn't already self-conscious or worried about the prospect of leaving him. I didn't need reminding! Nobody asked me how I was, it was always just how much did baby weigh.* Hayley Shing

It seems almost like a conspiracy, as we are all blind to it, and therefore cannot change it because we don't even know it's wrong. In the meantime, new mothers suffer.

> *I had my baby boy at 7.09am. I was home by 2.30pm and cooking dinner for the family at 5.30pm. I didn't even think it was wrong.* Michelle Bennett

> *One week after my emergency section I was told by my mother-in-law that I should 'get outside and walk in the*

fresh air', as it would do me and the baby good. I found it difficult to move from my bed to my sofa at this point. It made me feel like I was already failing as I couldn't get out and maybe I was depriving my baby of the 'fresh air'.
Gemma Bridges

When I was at home after my daughter's birth (it must have been a week or so after the birth) the midwife arrived for a visit when I was upstairs and as I came to the top of the stairs I heard her say to my husband 'Why is she in bed again? She's been upstairs every time I've called, she needs to be up and about!' I had had a caesarean and had been up and about, but remember feeling told off and also conflicted as I thought it would be ok and sensible to have a gentle start and rest when needed. Yvonne Hopkinson

As a society we fail to recognise that with every newborn baby comes a newborn mother, and she is just as tender and sensitive as the new baby. As a doula, I have found that most new mothers tend to be unaware that the support they get is lacking. They are grateful for the baby gifts or the bouquets of flowers, and it doesn't occur to them to ask for gifts that would be more useful, because they do not even know what their needs are. I worked for six years as an NCT antenatal teacher, and it has only occurred to me recently that while a great part of the course was focused on practical babycare, none of it was focused on the care of the new mother. I did run activities about the impact of the baby's arrival on the couple's relationship, and I talked about sleep deprivation and ways to manage it, and about what to expect in terms of body changes after the birth, but I had absolutely nothing on encouraging new mothers to see the postpartum as a major transitional phase, physically, emotionally and spiritually, and to think about what they might need during that period. Our total cultural lack of awareness is staggering.

Long before I was a parent or doula, my friend Anne, from Norway, came to stay at my house when her son was a few months old. Despite my lack of experience looking after babies (I had never changed a nappy!), I offered to look after him in the morning so she could have a lie-in. She burst into tears and said that I was the first person to offer to do that for her, and not even her own mother had done so.

Our culture also glorifies the new mother who 'gets her life back' as soon as possible, and there is immense pressure to go out and 'look normal' and fit back into pre-pregnancy clothes. This too can result in feelings of inadequacy and shame.

Claire already had a 13-month-old daughter when she found herself pregnant with twins. Her pregnancy was complex medically, which meant that from 24 weeks onwards she was at the hospital twice a week for scans and check-ups. Her daughters were born at 32 weeks by emergency caesarean, then spent five weeks in NICU. When I met her they had only just come home and were being fed via a mix of breast and tube-feeding (which took over two hours, including feeding and pumping, leaving Claire with just a 30-minute break between feeds). I supported Claire as a postnatal doula, and I helped her put her twins in a stretchy wrap sling together for the first time. I asked if I could take a picture to share on social media with her permission (so that other twin mums knew it was possible to carry two babies together). Claire asked me to retake the picture, because, she said, 'I look fat'. This made me feel so sad. She had grown two brand-new humans, and was managing to feed them under very challenging conditions, but rather than celebrating the amazing thing she had achieved, she was worried about her figure. This is no judgement on Claire, because I remember worrying that I was fat after giving birth myself. But can you imagine how different women would feel if everyone around them reminded them to be gentle with themselves and their physical recovery, and showered them with compliments about how well they were doing?

My first child was a baby with very intense needs. He cried all day unless he was being held and rocked. I remember feeling utterly exhausted and lonely and struggling with guilt, because I thought I ought to feel 'fulfilled' by motherhood. As I walked in parks pushing the pram that he hated and in which he cried unless it was constantly moving, I remember seeing groups of new mums sitting together and feeling a deep sense of longing for adult company and friendship.

When people say 'enjoy every minute'. You are not going to enjoy every minute because we are human beings with ups and downs anyway, BUT the postnatal period is such a sacred time in terms of bonding, recovery, care of both mother and baby etc etc. All this horrible phrase does is pile expectations on new mums at a very vulnerable time when they may feel guilt/sadness etc when they don't enjoy every minute, which is totally OK and normal!
Sarah Stanhope

Besides the lack of appropriate support, new mothers are also inundated with well-meaning 'advice', which most of the time only serves to increase their feelings of inadequacy.

This book is a call to action to encourage you to reclaim the practice of lying-in and request support for your recovery. Traditionally lying-in was for about a month, so aiming towards this would be a fantastic goal. I appreciate how challenging it can be in our culture, however, so aiming for two weeks, or even a week, could still make an enormous difference to your and your family's wellbeing.

Remember: because you, as the mother, are vital to your family, making sure that you are looked after isn't selfish. Everybody benefits from a well mother: mother, baby, partner and other children.

Midwives tell me that women used to be encouraged to spend a week in the bed, and a week around the bed. Now I know this isn't right for many women, as they simply don't have enough support or would go stir crazy, but there is much to be gained by adapting this wisdom in the first month after the birth and having regular naps. Some mums nap with their baby in the morning and then again in the afternoon!

Remember your baby will benefit from this too, as you can spend more time getting to know her, doing skin-to-skin, establishing breastfeeding if that's how you are feeding and generally slowing down.

While in this book I mostly focus on the mother, because she is the one recovering from the amazing feat of growing and birthing another human, partners get a raw deal from the lack of support in our culture too. Most only get two weeks of paternity leave, which can often amount to less if labour lasts a few days, or the mother ends up staying in hospital after birth. Then, especially for a first baby, unless the mother has some family nearby, she might find herself alone at home all day with her baby, without a social network, because all her friends are working daytime jobs. This puts immense pressure on just one person, who is usually away all day, to provide the support that the new mother needs.

If few people ask the new mother how she is doing, even fewer ask the new father. There is also societal pressure for the new dad to 'be strong' and not show any 'negative' feelings. Yet the percentage of fathers experiencing postnatal depression is estimated to be between 4 and 25 percent (Kim and Swain, 2007).

In the early years of teaching antenatal classes, when my classes were eight evening sessions of two hours, I always had a 'women-only' class, and a 'fathers-only' class. I invited the other half of the class to go to the pub instead. I naively expected that the women would get more from the women-only class than their partners. I was very surprised to find the opposite. During the fathers-only class men would open up about their fears, and express all the stuff that they hadn't dared to say in front of their partners. I found the class to be incredibly positive and transformative for them.

I once heard about a new dad who was asked by a doula how he was, and burst into tears. He said 'Not even my own mother asked me that'.

What I have noticed is that after both births, no one ever asked how my partner was. Neil, after the first birth, was doing everything apart from breastfeed. He was running the house and changed every nappy. He looked after Henry as I hadn't bonded with him. He was mum, dad, my carer and full-blown cook and cleaner in the first one to two months. He was run ragged. But no one asked him how he was. Hannah Burns

Supporting partners, so that they can support mothers, can have positive effects on the family as a whole.

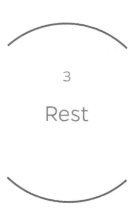

3

Rest

Have you ever done a 24-hour-a-day job before? Where you have to wake up every two hours? Without a break? Or any days off. And did you start this job immediately after undergoing a painful, major medical procedure? Where you might have lost a lot of blood, and/or been injected with prescription drugs? AND did this job involve a major, irreversible change in your role in life, with serious emotional ramifications? Kate Evans

Mothers cannot give from a depleted source. Every mother needs emotional, mental, physical, and spiritual validation, nourishment, and support. When a mother is respected and well cared for, she and her whole family will benefit. www.theearlydays.net

Of the four tenets of postnatal recovery, rest is probably the most important. Regardless of what research has to say, it should be common sense that when a woman has grown and birthed a baby, she should get a chance to rest and recover from the process.

When you think about all the classic pregnancy ailments, and about how tired pregnant women are during their third trimester (pregnancy is divided into trimesters, the first being from conception to three months, the second from four to six months, and the third from seven to nine months), and then that some women labour over several days without sleep, and may then end up with major abdominal surgery, it seems truly crazy that ensuring that she can rest and recover isn't standard practice and a matter of priority. Not to mention the fact that after the birth she is responsible for the survival of a vulnerable and needy infant.

If someone was scheduled to have abdominal surgery for any other reason, and was told 'Oh, and by the way, after your surgery you'll be looking after a tiny sleepless infant 24/7 and will need to wake up at least every two to three hours to feed it', you can be sure that person would say 'Are you crazy? That's not possible, I'll be recovering from major abdominal surgery!'. Even with a straightforward vaginal birth a new mother still desperately needs rest. This is why, traditionally, women have been supported by family members.

We all know about how exhausting new parenthood is, and there are many memes and jokes about new parents' sleep deprivation. However, there doesn't seem to be recognition of the fact that exhaustion isn't something to just to get on with. Extreme tiredness can be avoided, or at least minimised, if you have the right support.

According to one review of the literature 'Nearly 64% of new mothers are affected by fatigue during the postpartum period, making it the most common problem that a woman faces as she adapts to motherhood' (Badr et al, 2017), and another paper reports that 'As many as 46%-87% of new mothers report problems with tiredness or fatigue' (Kurth et al, 2010).

Interestingly, there is very little focus on rest from a maternity care point of view. Almost no mention is made of it in the NICE guidelines for postpartum care (NICE guideline CG37, 2006). There is a mention of the word fatigue, but it means pathological fatigue:

Fatigue 1.2.43 Women who report persistent fatigue should be asked about their general wellbeing, and offered advice on diet, exercise and planning activities, including spending time with her baby. [2006] 1.2.44 If persistent postnatal fatigue impacts on the woman's care of herself or baby, underlying physical, psychological or social causes should be evaluated. [2006] 1.2.45 If a woman has sustained a postpartum haemorrhage, or is experiencing persistent fatigue, her haemoglobin level should be evaluated and if low, treated according to local policy. [2006]

I believe that many new mothers would find some irony in the use of the words 'persistent fatigue'! The only mention of the word rest in the whole document is about the importance of it for establishing breastfeeding on the postnatal ward:

Where postnatal care is provided in hospital, attention should be paid to facilitating an environment conducive to breastfeeding. This includes making arrangements for: 24-hour rooming-in and continuing skin-to-skin contact when possible, privacy, adequate rest for women without interruption caused by hospital routine...

This is perhaps not surprising, as it reflects the lack of a holistic approach to medicine. When you go to the doctor because you are unwell, how often do they ask you how much sleep you are getting?

A literature search on the topic of postnatal rest did not find much. There are a handful of publications on postpartum fatigue, which is a reflection of research's tendency to assess treatment of symptoms rather than interventions that improve health in general. One paper states that: 'Postpartum fatigue is a very common complaint among postpartum women, with 88.5% of vaginal-birth women expressing this complaint in a recent study' (Hsieh et al, 2018).

From April 2020, an NHS initiative means that new mothers will receive a dedicated six-week check, to discuss their physical and mental health, which is separate from their baby's six-week check. This reinstates funding that was previously cut. I am pleased that the government sees the importance of taking into account the health and wellbeing of new mothers, and I would like to encourage you to be open with your healthcare provider if you aren't OK, and to go back for further appointments if needed.

I would like to introduce you to the concept of preparing for rest before the birth. There are three reasons for this. First, just as it is easier to plan for birth options before you go into labour, so it is easier to plan for your postnatal recovery while you are not sleep deprived and trying to manage the intense needs of a newborn. Similarly, the point of a plan is not so much the plan itself, but rather the process of exploring and thinking through options. (More details on this in Chapter 8.)

Second, the way your birth unfolds may impact your recovery. While most of us understand that recovering from a surgical birth may take longer than from a vaginal one, it can be more complex than this. For example, on a physical level a mother may recover faster from a calm, planned caesarean than from a five-day long induction followed by an instrumental birth.

Thirdly, the rest you get before you give birth can also impact your recovery. When I was pregnant with my first child, who was due in early February, I stopped work before the Christmas holiday. I was originally planning to work longer, and I am grateful to the HR person who noticed how tired I was and encouraged me to stop earlier. My son was born two weeks after his due date, which meant that I had nearly two months of rest before his birth. I had a fantastic, relaxing time. I did it again when pregnant with my daughter, because it had worked so well for me the first time. I'm not alone; some other mums feel the same:

I stopped work the first time at 28 weeks because I knew I wasn't going to return to my job and had no interest in working for the sake of it when it was a very demanding time of year. The next two times I stopped around 28 weeks again. I just found that my body was completely slowing down and everything was an enormous effort and it felt wrong to push through it when my body was clearly asking me to listen. I don't know how people do it – working to the end... it felt impossible to me. Wendy Evans

I left the month before I was due. We could get by just fine without my pay because we had planned for that. It was great because I was sooo tired all the time. Megan EJ

I went on leave five weeks before my due date. Two weeks were holiday I had to take before. I had low blood pressure and polyhydramnios so the extra time was more than welcome. I don't regret a single nap. I was induced at 38 weeks in the end so I'm even more glad I took some time to rest and fill the freezer with batch-cooked meals.

Looking back with hindsight it was lovely to have some time just for me as well before life changed to the new 24/7 in demand role. I love my boy with everything I am, but little snippets of time just for me are bliss too. Emma Aldous

In France, the maternity leave system makes it obligatory to stop work six weeks before the due date. When I started working as a doula, I was shocked that in the UK women work right up until their due date. Once, a client actually went into labour at work.

I think there are two issues here. Firstly, first-time mothers are often asked to book their time off during their second trimester, when they have no idea how tired they'll be in their third trimester. Secondly, either maternity leave isn't long enough, or women want to keep all their maternity leave for after their baby is born. This is understandable, but it also shows how our culture is skewed to focus on the idea that only the baby matters, and that taking time for yourself is somehow selfish.

My instinct told me that doing nothing before the birth was important. In an article entitled 'The last days of pregnancy, a time in between', midwife Jana Studelska talks about the importance of this time:

I believe that this is more than biological. It is spiritual. To give birth, whether at home in a birth tub with candles and family or in a surgical suite with machines and a neonatal team, a woman must go to the place between this world and the next, to that thin membrane between here and there. To the place where life comes from, to the mystery, in order to reach over to bring forth the child that is hers. The heroic tales of Odysseus are with us, each ordinary day. This round woman is not going into battle, but she is going to the edge of her being where every resource she has will be called on to assist in this journey.

We need time and space to prepare for that journey. And somewhere, deep inside us, at a primal level, our cells and hormones and mind and soul know this, and begin the work with or without our awareness.

I researched the topic of antenatal rest in the scientific literature. As the authors of one study state, there is very little research into the effect of antenatal leave on birth outcome. And as the authors of another study say, 'Maternity leave policies are presumed to be essential to ensure the health of pregnant workers and their unborn children. However, little is known about the optimal duration of prenatal maternity leave and existing policies are not evidence-based' (Hammer et al, 2018). It appears that the effect of antenatal leave on post-birth outcomes (for instance, postpartum fatigue) has not been studied at all.

The handful of studies that exist seem to draw a link between the length of antenatal maternity leave and birth outcomes. In one paper (Guendelman et al, 2009), the authors studied women who either took maternity leave early or who worked right up until they gave birth. They found that women who took leave were almost four times less likely to have a caesarean birth than those who worked until they gave birth. Similarly, the authors of a Canadian study found a correlation between those who worked right up until the birth, and the rate of complications during labour. They found that women who had a straightforward birth had, on average, taken a week more of antenatal maternity leave than the women who had complications during their birth (Xu et al, 2002). However, this is not the full picture. Some studies took place in the US, where there is no legal paid maternity leave in the majority of states and women often have no choice in the matter, and one paper actually linked antenatal maternity leave to poorer birth outcomes, because these women had unhealthy pregnancies (Goodman et al, 2017). Overall the lack of research highlights the fact that our culture has little understanding of how important the perinatal period is.

I don't blame women for not taking leave early enough to give themselves time to rest before they give birth. I know that many women work until they give birth because they have no choice, often for economic reasons. I feel that the blame should rest squarely on a culture that fails to understand and support the needs of birthing women, rather than on women themselves. I also know that each woman is different and has different needs, and that for some a long break before birth could actually have detrimental effects.

With my first, I finished work 10 weeks before she came along and on reflection, I regret it a huge amount. I didn't have many friends locally and my own family were 300 miles away; I was struggling with a family loss in recent months at the time and those 10 weeks allowed my anxiety to set in, too much time on my hands to just sit and think... And overthink... and overthink some more.
Danielle Cooke

First I had some annual leave to use, so from about 30 weeks I took Wednesdays off and that worked well. I started maternity leave at 36 weeks – helped remove our old kitchen before the new kitchen was installed. My hypnobirthing teacher told me there'd be time to paint the kitchen after baby arrived. I think she was just trying to get me to slow down (the kitchen painting didn't get finished for a couple of years). Birthed baby at 40+6.

What would I do differently? Well I know much more now, but had no idea at the time, plus I operated by keeping busy, achieving practical tasks. I had anxiety but no tools to acknowledge and deal with it. Corinne Rooney

With this discussion I would like to encourage women, and birth workers, to consider the idea that some women may really benefit from building in some time to rest before their due date.

When it comes to rest after the birth, the NICE guidelines for postnatal care do say that 'Women should be offered relevant and timely information to enable them to promote their own and their babies' health and wellbeing and to recognise and respond to problems', and that 'At each postnatal contact, women should be asked about their emotional wellbeing, what family and social support they have and their usual coping strategies for dealing with day-to-day matters'. However, in practice I do not see this happening. The system is simply too stretched, and midwives, maternity support workers and health visitors do not have enough time to facilitate this type of discussion. This isn't a criticism of health professionals, who I know work tirelessly and do their best. I would like to see maternity health professionals bringing up the idea of the importance of rest with families before the birth, when there is perhaps a little more time to explore the idea.

My experience as an antenatal teacher and doula has shown that there are several issues with our culture when it comes to postnatal rest. First, we have abnormal expectations about what the postpartum period looks like: the media tends to show us new babies dressed in pristine white, peacefully sleeping. This contributes to an unhealthy expectation of the realities of parenthood. When I taught antenatal classes, I used to tell new parents that during the first six weeks, if they got washed, dressed, and fed themselves and the baby, it was a good day!

Another problem is that our culture encourages independence and individualism over interdependence and collectivism (Small, 1998). In this context, the ability to care for oneself, alone, with no support, is seen as a sign of strength. This is one of the reasons that 'getting back to normal' is seen as so desirable. This belief is so ingrained, and yet so unconscious, that it can lead new mothers to feel guilty about having or needing support. In *The Golden Month*, Jenny Allison explains:

Letting go of independence can be a challenge, especially when we are brought up with the consistent message of how highly prized it is. Even though someone from outside the Western culture might not understand why a mother would insist on her independence at this time (in a life of hard work, why not ask for help when you can?), it also depends on those around you to give you permission to feel entitled. So this part is not always so easy to do for mothers in the West.

Furthermore, this 'independence', which makes rest more challenging for new mothers, leads to an abnormal expectation of independence in newborn babies, along with the idea that we will spoil them if we meet their needs, or 'create a rod for our own back'. This is misguided, because we have over 60 years of research (since John Bowlby came up with the theory of attachment) to disprove this idea and show that the opposite occurs: babies whose needs for closeness and comfort are met grow up to be happier and more confident adults than those whose needs were ignored (Gerhardt, 2004).

We are a carrying species, so human infants protest when they are separated from us. Even when deeply asleep, our babies sense when they are put down and wake up and cry. This, and our unrealistic cultural expectation that babies should sleep for long periods on their own, creates unnecessary stress and contributes to new parents' fatigue. If you'd like to read more on the topic, the BASIS (Baby Sleep Information Source) website is a fantastic, evidence-based resource, as is the book *Sweet Sleep* by La Leche League.[*]

One way to meet your baby's need for contact and closeness, and your own need to get around and fix yourself a snack, is to get a baby carrier. I was once the mother of a 'velcro baby' who refused to be put down, and this led me to become a babywearing instructor and trainer. The evidence for the use of a sling for both parents and babies is compelling. Aside from the fact that it gives you your hands back, your baby is likely to be calmer: carried babies cry on average 40 percent less (Hunziker and Barr, 1986) and are calmed by being carried (Esposito et al, 2013). Many parents find that being able to meet their baby's needs more easily builds confidence and feelings of wellbeing and competence, as well as conserving energy by not having to 'fight' against a baby who protests every time they try to put them down. You can even use a sling for daytime sleep www.basisonline.org.uk/using-a-sling-for-daytime-sleep.

There are many styles of baby carrier. Choosing a sling is a bit like choosing a pair of jeans. What suits your friend may not suit you. Ergonomics is key and will make the difference between something that you can comfortably use for hours and something that may cause you backache within a few minutes! There are now plenty of sling consultants and sling libraries and drop-ins around the country, and it's well worth investing in professional support to help you choose the right sling for you. You can find a local consultant or library at www.slingpages.co.uk. Carrying Matters is a brilliant resource www.carryingmatters.co.uk. And if you want to read more on

---

[*] You can find links to this and many other useful resources on my website: sophiemessager.com

the topic, I recommend Rosie Knowles' *Why Babywearing Matters* in this series (Pinter & Martin, 2016).

One thing that I've found difficult, as a doula and antenatal educator, is conveying the reality of new parenthood to expectant parents without being alarmist, while still trying to be realistic. This is tricky, because everyone's experience will be completely different. When I taught NCT classes, in the same class reunion session I often had couples who asked 'Why didn't you tell us it would be so hard?', while in the same group I would have parents who found it easier than they expected.

One good way to look at it, which helps you think flexibly, is to consider your own values and how you like to be in control of your life, and view your baby as a new guest in your house. When someone comes to stay with you for the first time, you don't know what their preferences are, so you try to enquire about things like dietary needs. Your new baby is just the same, but because you can't ask them about their preferences before they arrive, it is useful to try and keep a flexible mindset.

I once supported a new mum who asked me in desperation if I had a magic wand to fix dinner time. Every evening she and her partner tried to settle their new baby daughter to sleep at 7pm in her cot upstairs so that they could relax as a couple and enjoy their dinner together. However, their daughter wouldn't settle by herself, and they spent the whole evening running up and down the stairs, unable to cook properly or eat together. I explained that I didn't have a magic wand, but that some parents choose to have the baby with them in a Moses basket or in a sling, or breastfeeding at the dinner table, and take turns eating while one is holding the baby. Some couples completely change the timing of their evenings and eat dinner much earlier. There are never quick fixes, but if you can look at the 'problem' creatively (tricky when sleep-deprived, I know), you can try out different ways of doing things that might work for you.

I say 'problem', because what is a problem for one person won't be for another. A new mother I supported wanted a one-off postnatal doula session to discuss sleep. I asked her to describe the problem. She said she would breastfeed her baby to sleep, then spend most of her evening going up and down every 45 minutes or so to resettle her. I asked if that bothered her and she said no. I was surprised, so I asked what the problem was. She said that everybody else was telling her that what she was doing was wrong. I gently explained that it was only a problem if it bothered her.

Because mothering isn't valued in our culture, another thing that can stop new mothers from resting (as well as depleting their mental energy) is that many feel guilty about 'doing nothing' all day when they are looking after a new baby. As a society we fail to see that mothering is no mean feat. Naomi Stadlen's wonderful book, *What Mothers Do: especially when it looks like nothing* (2004) expresses it very well:

> *Most people would say that rinsing baby clothes meant that she was working, whereas picking up her baby meant that she had to spend a lot of time not working. Mothers frequently describe a painful sense of 'failure' about exactly those moments, when if we look closer, we notice that they were mothering their babies. The reverse is also true. When a mother is rushing around, busy with household tasks, that may be concrete and visible, but are surely much more peripheral to the work of being a mother, both she and other people are likely to say that she is 'managing to get her work done'.*

Another article (Rust, 2020) explains it well too:

You will not get anything done when you are home with a baby. And anyone who told you otherwise is not being very forthcoming (or perhaps they just have a lousy memory). So what are you doing all day? Not much that can be measured, really.

You're simply responding appropriately and with patience (through fatigue) to smiles, to tears, to hunger cues and to drowsiness, teaching your baby how to navigate this complex and (to a baby) highly emotional and raw world.

Helping new mothers to see the incredible value of their mothering is very important.

I'm also aware that, to be able to relax, a new mum needs *some* tasks to be done. As a postnatal doula, when I meet new parents before the birth and they ask me what I do, I often say this: there is usually one task, be it the laundry, or having no dirty dishes in the sink, that will bother you a lot if it's not done. That's one task I'll make sure to do for you. You can also do this yourself if you don't have a doula, because there is a lot to be said for dropping your standards for a while in the early weeks after the birth. If you can think about what would really bother you if it wasn't done, and plan to do that and only that, you may find it easier to ignore the stuff that bothers you less.

Some suggestions you could put in place to ensure you are get enough rest after birth

The suggestions listed below are by no mean exhaustive, or rules to be followed. They are ideas and examples, and may help you think about what might work in your circumstances.

- Organise as much support as possible ahead of time.
- Try and keep early afternoons free for napping, which is when most of us are at our sleepiest.
- Make a note for the door to avoid being woken up during your nap by unwanted visitors. Something like 'New mother and baby sleeping, please don't knock or ring the doorbell. Leave deliveries by the door/in this safe place/come back later'.
- Think of ways to get chores like cooking, buying food, cleaning and doing laundry done so you can rest. All these things tie into one another.
- Consider writing a postnatal recovery plan to help you explore your options and communicate what you'd like to your friends and family. This is easier to do before the birth.
- Make a list of all the possible support people that could come and help you get some rest after the birth. Explain ahead of time what you will be trying to achieve, and ask for specific help from people. People love to help, but often they don't know how to. Choose your supporters wisely: ideally they should be both helpful and make you feel good. Having someone bossy who irritates you won't help you rest, and nor will someone who expects to be waited on. While support is important, so is the fact that the new mother feels both supported and firmly in the driving seat.
- If you can afford it, consider hiring a postnatal doula. Or get family and friends to buy you doula vouchers. This can be a game-changer (more in Chapter 7).

Alleviating the pressure of running a household is an important part of getting postnatal rest. Support from your partner is essential, and research shows that the first cause of disputes in couples after the birth of a baby is 'who does what'. You might like to try this activity with your partner if you have one, or you can do it by yourself.

- Sit down with your partner if you have one.
- Separately write a list of all the chores and who does them (separately because this exercise might show that you have difference perceptions of who does what).
- Try to be as comprehensive as possible and write everything down, including things that only happen seasonally like mowing the lawn.
- Sit down and compare notes.

As the new mother, especially if she is breastfeeding, will be doing the brunt of the babycare, see what tasks can be dumped, outsourced, or taken on by your partner. You can use a similar model to try and plan for the multitude of new tasks a newborn baby brings, such as nappy changing and extra laundry, and explore whether you have different expectations about the split of tasks. If you'd like to read more, the book *Baby's here! Who does what?* is useful and easy to read (Fisher, 2010), and Graeme Seabrook has an online course called Motherload Liberation (www.graemeseabrook.com). If you'd like to explore in more depth how having a newborn can impact your relationship with your partner, with wonderful creative solutions, try the book *Becoming Us* (Taylor, 2011), which has a website and online course too (becomingusfamily.com).

When it comes to rest, you may have heard the expression 'sleep when the baby sleeps'. While it's sometimes bandied around in an unhelpful manner, there is some wisdom in it. What I've observed, however, is that it's quite common for new mothers to feel guilty about what they are not doing, so as soon as the baby drops off, they run around trying to do everything.

I think this is quite normal behaviour when you are coping with the change that a new baby brings: you try to do things like you did before. But it doesn't really work, and often creates more tiredness and stress.

The more you can take it easy and lie down with your baby the better, even if you don't sleep. This can help keep visitors in the frame of mind to look after you, instead of the other way round. Consider holding your baby skin-to-skin while you are lying down. While this has great benefits for your baby, it also has benefits for you. Babies held skin-to-skin cry less, but it can also promote rest as you can justify lying down in bed as an activity that is good for your baby. The release of feel-good hormones in your brain will facilitate bonding, and help with lactation (Hansford, no date). In fact, the authors of a review on skin-to-skin state:

> *Skin-to-skin contact stimulates the release of oxytocin, which antagonizes the fight-or-flight response, decreases anxiety, and increases calmness and social responsiveness. This may contribute to a physiological state that is more conducive to effective parenting.* (Cleveland et al, 2017)

What if you find it hard to nap during the day? Your baby has finally fallen asleep. So you think 'Right, I *must* go to sleep now', and you lie in bed restlessly, much as you would if you went to bed early knowing you had to get up at 4am. Often you end up wakeful and frustrated, or you finally fall asleep ten minutes before the baby wakes up! The trick here is to make your goal *rest*, not sleep. Any lying down is good, even with a book. Some women find it helpful to listen to a guided meditation or relaxation soundtrack. Often, if you lie down planning to relax rather than sleep, sleep comes more easily.

I was once in a baby yoga class and we went around the

circle to say how our week had been. Each mother bemoaned the fact that their baby's sleep was terrible. When it got to me, I said 'Doesn't this tell us something? There is nothing wrong with our babies, it's just the way they are'. There is a lot of wisdom in not 'fighting' against the new normal and wasting energy trying to change things that cannot be changed. If you can accept that things will get better even if you do nothing, as your baby grows, and put strategies in place to manage for yourself as best as you can in the meantime, it will help you to cope. For some mothers this means going to bed really early (as in, with the baby) a few times a week, while for others it means that their partner gets up early and takes the baby, so they can have an extra hour in bed.

Do consider co-sleeping. I know that it has bad press, because public health messages in the past led both health professionals and parents to believe that it is dangerous. However, research shows otherwise: when certain safety rules as followed, co-sleeping is as safe as sleeping on a different surface. In the La Leche League book *Sweet Sleep,* which covers the subject in depth, there is a checklist, the 'Safe Sleep 7' to use as a guideline. If you are:

1. a non-smoker
2. sober and unimpaired
3. a breastfeeding mother and your baby is
4. healthy and full-term
5. on his back
6. lightly dressed and you both are
7. on a safe surface

then your baby in bed with you is at no greater risk of SIDS (Sudden Infant Death Syndrome) than if he's nearby in a crib. The guidelines from the Lullaby Trust, a cot-death charity, have recently been changed to reflect this. If you'd like to read more, the BASIS website is a fantastic evidence-based resource by Durham University.

The evidence also shows that co-sleeping mothers get more sleep (McKenna, 2007). A co-sleeping baby can stir and almost wake up when she needs to feed, but since she is right next to her mother, the mother can breastfeed or soothe her back to sleep before she fully wakes up. Breastfeeding during the night is also easier when baby is nearby, because you don't have to fully rouse yourself and get out of bed to pick your baby up, and you don't have to soothe her back to sleep afterwards.

I know that co-sleeping isn't right for some families, and that's OK. But you might not know whether it will benefit you or not until you try it. Some new mothers tell me that they find it hard to sleep with a baby in their bed, and sometimes it's simply because it's the same as sleeping with a new partner. It takes some getting used to. It's also not an all-or-nothing thing. You may choose to co-sleep just for tonight, or for one nap, when you are desperate for some rest. It doesn't mean that you have to commit to it for the rest of your life. Talking things through with a doula or experienced co-sleeping parent can help.

Here are some stories from mums who planned ahead to make sure they would get some rest after they gave birth.

I hired professional post-natal home care – kraamzorg, in Belgium. They did my laundry, light shopping, my meals, and took care of my baby while I slept. It's allowed up to three months after birth; they were kind to extend a bit, as our baby had reflux. Pricing depends on the income level, so government steps in to make these services more available. I was very lucky. Otherwise, no grandparents living or able to help, no family living nearby. I started to think about it because I paid for post-natal services, I've got no free help otherwise. Laura Linde

The best thing for postnatal recovery was great access to excellent support via my midwife, doulas, breastfeeding specialists and lactation consultants (when needed). That allowed me to deal with the milk blebs, nearly getting mastitis, and her tongue tie and feel supported and safe throughout. Jo Evershed

The way I planned my postnatal care was: birth doula; postnatal doula; placenta encapsulation; closing the bones ceremony; belly-wrapping; babywearing; co-sleeping; expressing breastmilk; a cleaner!! Making a conscious effort to eat and drink well. The belly-wrapping has been absolutely key to starting to become mobile around the house, and having a postnatal doula has been incredible. She has made me feel loved, cared for and relaxed. I am also following my cultural practice of 40 days transition period where my I keep my baby indoors for 40 days. She will have time to adjust and transition from womb to world. I keep her warm and she mostly stays in my bedroom. I am feeding on demand and she sleeps in bed with me. I am sleeping during the day when she sleeps which I never did with my first two. I am taking regular Epsom salt baths and allowing the house to be a complete mess! Seema Barua

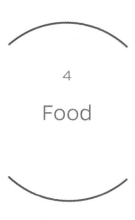

4

Food

There are three main requirements from the diet after delivery. To replace lost blood and nutrients, to repair damaged tissues and heal the uterus and vagina, and to support breastfeeding. There is a fourth requirement also which is that food provides a source of warmth for the body. Jenny Allison

In the first precious days following birth, your awareness is so intent on the baby that you may neglect your own needs. You will heal faster and be equipped to be an even better mother if you get enough rest, eat nutritious food often, drink plenty of healthful fluids, and get lots of help. Robin Lim

It seems like common sense that good nutrition should be essential for the optimal recovery of the new mother. Even Western science recognises that growing and birthing a baby (and feeding) depletes a mother's nutrients (Serralach, 2018).

Traditional wisdom has always acknowledged this, and cultural practices across the globe include wholesome recipes to nourish new mothers. Certain foods are encouraged to promote healing and restore health, and so are certain herbs or tonics. Most cultures also have dietary restrictions, because the prohibited foods are believed to cause illness either immediately or at a later stage in life. The most common is the avoidance of cold foods and drinks, both in the literal and the energetic sense (Dennis, 2007).

We all know that warming, nourishing recipes, such as chicken soup, are traditionally given to convalescent people, and that when we feel weak or unwell we crave these warming, comfort foods. It makes sense that they should be given to new mothers too. Obviously pregnancy and birth are not an 'illness', but seeing a new mother as someone who is in recovery, and treating her as such, means that visitors are more likely to bring gifts of food. What is more comforting than a hearty, home-cooked meal?

When I was pregnant with my first child, I met a lovely American couple, Suzanne and Bob, during antenatal classes. Suzanne unexpectedly went into labour at 32 weeks, and their baby daughter Olivia ended up having a long stay in the hospital neonatal unit. I went to visit Suzanne there, and I took her homemade beef stew. A couple of years ago – about 12 years after the birth of her daughter – Suzanne told me that she still remembers that I was the only person who brought her a casserole, and how much it meant to her.

When I gave birth to my second child, I hired independent midwives Siobhan Taylor and Amy Sutton. As part of their service, they provided three days of home-cooked meals. Despite being second-time parents and feeling more competent than after the birth of our first child, I still remember how special those meals were. The first food I ate after giving birth was a delicious fruitcake that Siobhan had baked for me. I also remember Amy bringing us the most amazing chicken pie and mash. The whole family benefitted from this, not just me and my husband and new baby, but also my three-year-old son, who spent a long time saying that 'midwives bring mashed potatoes'. There is something very special, nurturing and comforting about food that's been cooked with love especially for you.

Many new mums have told me that they remember fondly the cakes and meals they were given after birth:

I still clearly remember the meal my neighbour (already a mum) gave to us: creamy chicken and broccoli bake. It really felt like soul food because she made it for giving to us. Corinne Rooney

A friend who is from Malaysia brought round a chicken stir fry with noodles and it was something that could be reheated easily. It was delicious and she explained that it was also to help with my qi which is low after birth and a reason why they cook in sesame oil, to help recover it. Abby Hopewell

The first meal my husband cooked and served after birth. It was quite ordinary but the best meal I've ever had: goulash with noodles and broccoli. Sonia Sampaolo

Your Groaning Cake! It's almost enough to make me want to get pregnant again. Heather Nedzynski

As each culture has a different diet, and therefore different recommendations, and because each family's needs are different, I am not going to provide a rigid list of dishes, but I want to give you some ideas and encourage you to think ahead about how you're going to get good food inside you after your baby is born.

There are certain basic principles common to postpartum diet practices around the world. The food is usually high in carbs, protein, good fats and iron, and full of warming spices and flavour. When we are recovering from something we usually fancy warm, comfort foods from our childhood. Simple things that spring to mind include porridge, soups, stews and pies. In a paper on traditional postpartum practices in China, the authors found that 'Categorised against Western medical standards, several zuo yuezi practices are beneficial, including eating more, eating protein rich food' (Raven et al, 2007). I'm a big believer in instincts, so follow your cravings and eat what takes your fancy, remembering that nutrient-dense food, rather than junk, will both satisfy you and help you recover. Here are some things new mums have told me they loved:

*Black pudding on a toasted English muffin with ketchup. I had it every day for two weeks.** Sophie Christophy

My mum made me Malaysian laksa, Penang style, every time. I had a bowl for a few days and it's very rich in iron. It was sublime! Azeeta Nielsen

My Ecuadorian mother-in-law made me quinoa soup! Was sooo good! Carly Lokrheim

Soup! Warming, nourishing, can be drunk one-handed from a cup. Tomato, lentil and spinach was a winner. Steph Kidd

---

* I found this surprising at first, but it makes sense as it's a very iron rich food, with 6.4mg per 100mg versus 2.4mg for steak.

I absolutely loved the jasmine rice porridge from the book
The First Forty Days *and it is my comfort breakfast to*
this day when I am feeling physically or emotionally low.
Rosie Dhoopun

The NICE guidelines on maternal and child nutrition cover supplements like folic acid and vitamin D, as well as issues like weight, but sadly don't include a section about what to look for in terms of good nutrition.

For guidance on how to eat a balanced diet, First Steps Nutrition Trust is an independent public health nutrition charity that provides evidence-based information. They have a resource called 'Eating Well for New Mums' that you can download free. There is an infographic on what a balanced diet might look like, options for vegetarians, what is useful in each food group, some tips on managing to eat well when you are a new mum and sample menus, recipes and suggestions for healthy snacks. There is also information on eating well while breastfeeding, supplements and special diets like dairy free, vegan and vegetarian.

Over the years I have developed a handful of favourite recipes to make for new mothers. One of these is the 'groaning cake'. I came across the recipe in a book called *The Birth House* (McKay, 2010), which is the story of a traditional midwife in Nova Scotia in the mid-1900s. The author explains:

The tradition of the groaning cake, or kimbly at (or following) a birth is an ancient one. Wives' tales say that the scent of a groaning cake being baked in the birth house helps to ease the mother's pain. Some say if a mother breaks the eggs while she's aching, her labour won't last as long. Others say that if a family wants prosperity and fertility, the father must pass pieces of the cake to friends and family the first time the mother and baby are churched (or the first time they go to a public gathering) after a birth. Many cultures share similar traditions... a special dish, bread, or drink, spiced with cinnamon, all spice, and/or ginger. At one time there was even a groaning ale made to go with it...

I have since discovered that the tradition originated from the UK, and that the postpartum period was called 'the groaning'. According to Victoria Williams, the word groaning 'was used to refer to the time extending from when a mother-to-be took to her bed to give birth, to the moment she became strong enough to walk around normally – that this period was called the groaning is a candid reference to women's labour pains' (Williams, 2016). The foods served included the cake, but also groaning cheese, pies, beer and wine. The cake was also used for pain relief, and the Cambridgeshire version included gin and hemp seed. The groaning cheese originated from Oxfordshire and was a large wheel of cheese, which was eaten starting from the middle. Once it was hollowed out, the baby was passed through the cheese for good luck (culturecheesemag.com/cheese-bites/groaning-cheese).

I bake a groaning cake before I go on call for a birth. I like to share the cake with the new parents and the midwife/birth team, which has earned me the nickname of the 'cake doula'. I also take one to my postnatal clients. The cake is moist and full of warming spices. The black treacle makes it an ideal postpartum food as it is rich in bioavailable iron. I have adapted the recipe slightly, and you can find gluten free, vegan, paleo and even keto versions on my blog.

Groaning cake

- 2½ cups (325g) flour
- 3 eggs
- 4tsp baking powder
- ½ cup (110ml) oil
- ½ cup(118ml) fresh orange juice
- 1tbsp mixed spice
- ¼ cup (90g) black treacle (I like to use ½ cup)
- 1⅓cups (260g) brown sugar
- 1½ cups (approx 100g) grated apple
- 1tsp vanilla extract
- 1tsp almond extract

Sift dry ingredients together. Add eggs, oil, orange juice, black treacle and sugar. Add almond and vanilla extract. Mix well. Add grated apple. Mix well. Pour into lined and greased loaf tins. Bake at 180°C (160°C if using a fan oven) for 35-40 minutes or until a skewer comes out clean. This recipe makes two loaves.

Another favourite recipe of mine (because of my husband's heritage) is chicken and red date soup. It's a Chinese take on traditional chicken soups made in the West. As well as the broth from the chicken being full of nutrients that are good for the new mother, Chinese medicine states that red dates are known to increase qi (life energy), and help nourish the blood and bring relaxation. The ginger, red dates and goji berries are considered to be warming to the body. I use a slightly modified version of the one found in Heng Ou's book *The First Forty Days*.

Chicken and red date soup

- 2lb whole chicken or chicken portions (I like to use thighs as they are easier to shred than drumsticks, it's best if they have bones)
- 1 onion, peeled
- 2in fresh ginger, peeled and halved
- 3 medium carrots, peeled and thinly sliced
- 5 Chinese red dates (you can find these online or in Asian supermarkets. Normal dates do not have the same medicinal properties)
- 3tbsp dried goji berries
- salt to taste

Place the chicken in a medium pot, and add enough cold water to cover the meat. Bring to a boil over medium-high heat, uncovered. Once boiling, add the onion and ginger. Season to taste. Reduce the heat to medium, cover, and cook for 40 minutes. Remove the lid occasionally to skim any foam off the top and discard. Remove from the heat. Move the chicken to a plate to cool. Shred the chicken meat with two forks. Place 1 to 2 cups of the shredded chicken back in the pot. Add the carrots and dates, and simmer over low heat, uncovered, for 45 minutes. Add the goji berries and cook an additional 15 minutes. Season with salt to taste.

I have found that I can make this soup more quickly in my Instant Pot (or you could use a normal pressure cooker). The recipe, plus links to scientific articles about the advantages of using red dates and goji berries, are on my blog.

It may be a good idea to invest in kitchen equipment such as an Instant Pot or slow cooker, or to ask for one as a gift or borrow from a friend for a few weeks. Then you can chuck ingredients in when you have time, and benefit from a warm meal later on without having to stay near the stove. Similarly, a rice cooker cooks rice to perfection without you having to keep an eye on it, and keeps it warm without overcooking for hours.

Another staple which is both quick to make and nourishing is fried rice. It's best done using cold, leftover rice, as freshly cooked rice will be too sticky.

Fried rice

- 3 cups (about 600g) of cold cooked rice
- A handful of frozen peas (you could use any chopped green veg)
- A handful of chopped spring onions (optional, as it works well without it too and you might not have time to chop stuff)
- A handful of bacon bits, leftover bits of chicken, small pieces of ham, or any other bits of meat you happen to have
- 1 egg

Heat a wok or frying pan over medium heat until very hot. Add a tablespoon of vegetable oil. Fry the meat and vegetables for a couple of minutes or until cooked through. Add the egg, stir well to scramble it. Add the rice and stir well. Cook until the rice is piping hot. Serve with sauces of your liking such as soy, chilli oil or sweet chilli sauce.

When I was a child, often on a Sunday evening, my mother would cook something she called a '*migouri*', using rice and whatever leftover meat and veg happened to be in the fridge. I have very fond memories of eating this dish, which was warm and comforting. The recipe above could also be made using pulses instead of rice, or leftover pasta, and spices of your choice.

Breakfast-wise, porridge or oatmeal is a great option for both comfort and the fact that oats are known to boost milk supply (Bonyata, 2017). But because new mothers often don't have the time to cook or make something nutritious, you could consider making overnight porridge (mix oats with milk and toppings of your choice, such as dates or dried apricots, which will help with gut transit as well as boosting iron), then leave in the fridge overnight so the oats swell. Heat it up in the microwave before eating, or enjoy it cold.

Another quick and easy breakfast option is to make a smoothie. However, smoothies are usually cold, and since we know that warm foods can be beneficial to new mothers, I'd like to introduce you to the idea of making a warm smoothie instead. I can imagine how lovely it would have been to be given one when I was stuck under a new baby!

Warm oaty chocolate smoothie

- 1tbsp cocoa powder
- 240ml (1 cup) milk of your choice
- 3tbsp rolled oats
- ½ a ripe medium-sized banana
- 8 nuts of your choice (almond, hazelnuts, walnuts etc)
- 1tsp chia seeds (optional)

You could prep the dry ingredients and put them into the smoothie maker the night before. Pour the milk into a jug. Microwave until warm (you can do this in a pan if you prefer). Place the oats, banana, hazelnuts, chia seeds, cocoa powder, and approx. a fifth of the milk mixture in your smoothie maker or blender. Add a bit of cold water if you think the liquid is too warm (check the instructions for your smoothie maker or blender, and make sure the liquid is warm, not hot, to avoid burning). Blend on high for about a minute, or until the liquid is smooth. Pour into a cup (an insulated one with a lid and handle will keep it warm when you get interrupted), and serve.

It's a good idea to have plenty of non-perishable, nutritious, easy to eat one-handed snacks like nuts and dried fruit around. You might also like some good quality chocolate. You may feel hungry, but be on your own and stuck under a feeding or sleeping baby. Some mothers like to make a feeding time snack 'hamper', which they keep next to where they feed their baby. This would be a lovely gift for a new mother.

Hydration is also paramount for wellbeing and recovery. It's very easy to become dehydrated when you're busy looking after a newborn. If you are breastfeeding you'll probably find that it makes you incredibly thirsty. I made sure there were sports-top bottles of water everywhere, including on each side of my pillow so I didn't have to twist my body while breastfeeding lying down! This also applies to when you're still in hospital, especially if you've had a caesarean and cannot move easily, and you are on your own, or the ward you are in doesn't allow partners to stay overnight. Some women have told me that they found this bottle called the hydrant very helpful as it can clip onto the hospital bed frame and has a handy tube that allows you to drink without moving (www.manageathome.co.uk/pd/the-hydrant-drinking-system_10389).

It is amazing how good a nice warm drink can make you feel when you're tired and frazzled, so you might want to get yourself a good-quality insulated mug with a handle, because when you have a new baby you never know when you'll get to drink that cup of tea you've made.

If you are looking for inspiration on postpartum meals, here is a list of resources.

Books

- *The First Forty Days*, Heng Ou. Chinese and Chinese fusion recipes, beautifully illustrated. There is a shopping list, and a handy 'cheat sheet'. Recipes include smoothies, porridge, broths, soups, stews, rice dishes, all-in-one meals called 'mother's bowls', puddings, snacks and drinks.
- *Nurturing New Families*, Naomi Kemeny. A recipe section at the end of the book includes a list of store-cupboard ingredients, snacks, and simple recipes like smoothies, soups, energy balls, cookies and cakes.
- *The Little Book of Self-Care for New Mums* has a section with tips for eating better, and recipes for breakfast, lunch and dinner, snacks and quick meals and teas.

Recipes for postpartum dishes and freezer meals

- lilynicholsrdn.com/real-food-postpartum-recovery-meals
- traditionalcookingschool.com/food-preparation/nourishing-postpartum-freezer-meals
- takethemameal.com

Frozen delivery meals

These companies offer vouchers so meals can be given as gifts.

- www.thefooddoula.co.uk
- www.cookfood.net

Ready to cook dishes

- www.hellofresh.co.uk
- www.gousto.co.uk

I also love the idea of 'meal trains'. In my village the local church organises two weeks of home-cooked meals for new parents this way. In *The Golden Month*, a woman who emigrated to New Zealand recreated a Dutch tradition of putting up a wooden stork outside the house to announce the birth, which started a new tradition of the stork being given to new families so that they would get food delivered (Allison, 2015). You could organise your own by asking people around you (there is even a website www.mealtrain.com), or better still get someone to organise it for you.

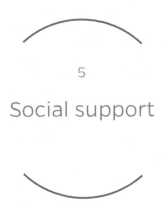

5

Social support

We don't have to do it all alone, we were never meant to.
Brené Brown

*When you study postpartum depression, there is a very
clear understanding that in communities where you see
more support, there is less depression.* Ariel Gore

As a new mother with my first child I felt extremely lonely. My
existing social network worked 9 to 5, and even though I pre-
empted this as much as I could by going to antenatal classes that
helped me meet other mums, the one mum I really bonded with
had a traumatic birth and couldn't get out for the first few weeks.
So for the first three months or so I was pretty much on my
own all day with my baby. I remember going for long walks and
looking longingly at groups of new mothers hanging out together
in parks. I struggled with feelings of shame and I didn't know
how to solve the problem. Eventually I met other mums at baby
classes, but I needed support earlier on and it just wasn't there.

Social support is an inherent part of your postpartum support. If you don't have people around you to support you, how will you rest, who will cook you food, keep your house tidy and look after other children? But beyond this, the mere presence of other adults around you as you find your way through motherhood has far-reaching effects beyond practical support. It is vital for your emotional wellbeing too.

If you feel lonely after birth, you aren't alone. According to some surveys, over 80 percent of new mums feel lonely (Packham 2017; Smith, 2018). Here is what some mothers said it was like for them:

I felt completely isolated in my early motherhood. Everything I knew about myself was turned on its head. Being a recent arrival to another country, people only knew me as a mother and I lost my frame of reference, making it incredibly hard to connect with anyone – other mums, my baby and most of all myself. I felt very alone and very ill at ease with it all. Laura Scarlett

Working in a male-dominated environment I was completely forgotten about while on maternity leave, not even one phone call in a whole 10 months. Couple that with living away from family and friends (military life has a lot of negative points) and my husband being deployed for the first three months of my youngest's life led to me developing an anxiety disorder, hardly leaving the house for six weeks. Rachael Ruddock

I was incredibly lonely after the arrival of my second. We moved area a couple of times, I had no established friends or support network, no local family and my husband worked full time. I think it was the loneliness and tiredness together that were the main triggers to me going

through my 'dark period'! It still gets to me now when I think back to that time, just how sad and lonely I really was. I think having friends and regular social interaction is an absolute must for any mum! Kelly Mitchell

I was on my own the day my husband went back to work. Having a baby really shows you who your real friends are: some stick with you, but a lot are lost on your journey to motherhood! I loved my baby but the days were monotonous and isolating and the sleep deprivation was harsh. I was eager to have a chat with anyone, the postman, window cleaner, checkout assistant in Sainsbury's. I longed for the moment my husband would come home from work and I'd have someone to talk to, before the loneliness of being up for half the night set in again. Kirstie Broughton

In her book *Mothering the New Mother*, Sally Placksin explains that:

Generations of women have been instructed that they would know how to mother because motherwit and the maternal instinct is a 'sacred calling' and birth rite. We all know how to do it; all we lack is the baby to put our innate talents into practice. But while mothers should be encouraged to trust their instincts (....) much of this mothering behaviour is learned not instinctive, and without the educational and emotional support of teachers and nurturers, it is much more difficult and stressful to master.

The difficulty with social isolation and loneliness is compounded by the fact that there is something very vulnerable about admitting to being lonely. You may experience feelings of shame, as if your lack of friends is a reflection of your lack of worth. Similarly, asking for help, in a culture that places such a high value on independence, can feel very challenging and as if you are failing.

I have seen so many new mothers struggle in silence because they believed they were the only ones finding it tough. There is societal taboo and silence around the struggles of motherhood that really needs to be broken. We need to change the narrative around the shame and silence, and help reclaim the postpartum support we used to have. Deep down, we know we aren't meant to be doing this alone. As part of the change, we need to embrace our need for support and be more open about our vulnerability.

> *Women experience a range of psychological stressors in the postpartum period. Social support has been shown to be effective in helping women cope with these stressors. Moreover, low levels or inconsistent social support have been found to be a strong predictor of postpartum depression.* (Negron et al, 2013)

Brené Brown is an American researcher who specialises in studying shame, and the power of vulnerability. As she explains, vulnerability isn't a weakness:

> *Vulnerability is the birthplace of love, belonging, joy, courage, empathy, and creativity. It is the source of hope, empathy, accountability, and authenticity. If we want greater clarity in our purpose or deeper and more meaningful spiritual lives, vulnerability is the path.* (Brown, 2015)

My hope is that if a small percentage of women start to demand support, it will spread and quickly become normal again. After all, 'set point theory' shows that it only takes 25 percent of the population to do something for it to rapidly become the new norm (Centola et al, 2018).

Another important aspect of societal support is whether it is genuinely supportive or judgemental. Unfortunately, our culture isn't supportive of new mothers, and it is often extremely judgemental. This really isn't helpful, because the majority of new mothers lack confidence as they navigate their new role. This is especially true for first-time mothers, who worry a lot about their mothering and whether they are 'good enough'. We need to boost new mothers' confidence. We need to remember that historically, even in the Western world, birth used to be a community and woman-centred event, and help was offered without people even having to ask (Placksin, 1998). Part of this support included boosting new mothers' self esteem, as explained in an account from a mother from Colombia:

> *People came to visit – the baby wasn't the centre of the whole thing. It was always the mother. The mother was always the centre – it was always 'Oh you did such a wonderful job' (...) She was praised, she was the centre, it was not like here in America, that the baby is everything and the mother is totally discarded and forgotten.* (Placksin, 1998)

I cannot stress enough the importance and power of confidence-boosting for the new mother. Many new mothers experience a lot of guilt. They doubt their own ability and worry that they aren't good enough as a mother. This is quite normal. But combine this with a culture in which almost every person the new mother encounters has some kind of 'advice' on how she ought to be raising her baby, and it is very easy for a new mother to feel that she is not doing a good job.

As a doula I always try and spot something positive, such as how tender and caring a mother is as she changes her baby, or how well she knows her baby's preferences, and acknowledge it. I have seen so many mothers burst into tears when I make simple positive statements like this. If you are visiting a new mother, I invite you to shift your focus, watch her closely, and notice when she does something you find lovely when she interacts with her baby. Then point it out.

Another aspect of societal support gone wrong is that women are silenced and unable to articulate their needs because society expects them to be ecstatic. I have lost count of the number of times a new mother has started telling me about not feeling good about her birth, and immediately followed it with the sentence 'But my baby is healthy and that's all that matters'. When women believe this, or are told this, it invalidates their feelings. When you feel wrong about feeling certain feelings, you cannot process them, or heal from them. Your feelings matter. You matter. Milli Hill, who started the Positive Birth Movement, explains:

When a woman gives birth, a healthy baby is absolutely completely and utterly the most important thing. It is not ALL that matters. Two things – just to repeat: a healthy baby is the most important thing, AND it is not all that matters. Women matter too. When we tell women that a healthy baby is all that matters we often silence them. We say, or at least we very strongly imply, that their feelings do not matter, and that even though the birth may have left them feeling hurt, shocked or even violated, they should not complain because their baby is healthy and this is the only important thing.

In my ten years working with new mothers, I have often been the first person to tell a mother that she has been lied to, and that her feelings matter.

When I tried to explain about the unkind treatment and choices that were wrongly denied to us during the first birth to my father-in-law, he cut me off mid-sentence and said 'But he's alright isn't he?'. He totally didn't want to hear anything about how it had emotionally affected me.
Hannah Burns

I think this is compounded by the fact that within Western culture, we aren't accustomed to sit with uncomfortable feelings, let alone with grief, so there is a tendency to look for the 'silver lining', because we mistakenly believe this to be helpful. However, research shows that this type of behaviour only results in the person feeling worse (because it implies that they are wrong for feeling the way they feel) as well as disconnected (because they do not feel understood). Here is an animated video on how to help a grieving friend that explains it in a very simple and clear way: www.refugeingrief.com/2018/07/19/help-a-friend-video.

I went to visit Kate, a new mother, to help her choose a sling. Her little girl had been born prematurely, and she had a traumatic birth, followed by a long stint in NICU and difficulties breastfeeding. I always ask about the birth, because it's important for me to know whether the birth might impact her body and therefore the support I offer. I also ask because I know how important it is to debrief birth experiences with someone who is listening with a non-judgemental, kindly ear. As Kate started telling me about the birth and early postnatal period, she became emotional and quickly stated that all that mattered was her daughter's health. I gently reframed it for her: 'It's OK to be happy that your daughter is healthy, and to feel crap about the birth and the experience around it, because these are two different things'. She burst into tears. I have had the same experience countless times when simply asking 'And how did that make you feel?' or saying 'I'm not surprised you're upset, because that sounds like a really tough experience'.

If you are visiting a new mother, I encourage you to ask these simple questions, listen carefully, and then gently validate and paraphrase whatever feelings you hear.

How to create a supportive network

While I know we often no longer live in close-knit communities, I believe it is possible to recreate, at least in part, some of the support women used to get. The most important thing you can do is to plan who can be there to support you after your baby is born. Who can support you practically, emotionally and with relevant information? This means support in your home, but also in the wider sense.

If you have a partner, it is worth sitting down and discussing your expectations of parenting and sharing the load before your baby arrives, because they might differ, and unspoken and unmet expectations can be the cause of unnecessary friction. Your partner might be your main source of support, but if they work in an employed capacity, they are likely to only get a couple of weeks leave, and you might be on your own with your baby for eight hours or more every weekday. Caring for a newborn is intense and demanding, and many new mothers desperately need a break when their partner comes home at the end of the day. When writing your postnatal recovery plan, include everybody who can support you, including your partner, but make sure to include as many other people as possible, because relying too much on one person is unlikely to provide you with enough support.

While ideally you'd have live-in help (or daily visits) for a while, anybody who can be an extra pair of hands for a couple of hours, bring you a casserole, run errands, shop, do a load of laundry or walk your dog would be valuable. Cast your net as wide as you can, from family to friends and acquaintances, work colleagues, and other mums who aren't newly postpartum themselves.

It is also worth trying to establish a postpartum support network of new parents going through the same thing at the same time, because although they might not be able to support you practically, they will be able to provide emotional support, as they will really understand what you're going through. One way to do this is to attend antenatal classes, whether childbirth preparation classes or antenatal exercise classes such as yoga, aquanatal or pilates.

The main reason couples say they book onto small-group antenatal classes is to meet other parents. This is valid for second-time parents too. As an antenatal class facilitator I put a lot of effort into helping to build the group beyond the class itself: I would ask someone to be a social secretary for the group and to organise a meal out before the babies' arrival. The feedback later stressed how helpful it was to have someone answer questions on the WhatsApp group at 3am and how reassuring it was to meet weekly for coffee mornings. Many people stay friends for years afterwards. It is worth finding out, ahead of time, what classes, drop-ins, and mother and baby groups there are in your area that you might want to visit.

If you establish and build your network of support before you baby arrives, it will be much easier than after the birth, when all your time will be taken by your new baby. If you're a first-time mum you may not know where to find local support, so connecting with mothers of slightly older children locally can be helpful.

I know it can be daunting to visit new groups as a new mum. You might feel worried or vulnerable. As a doula I have sometimes accompanied new mothers on a first visit to a local mother and baby group. Having someone you know a little, even if only from online chats, could make a world of difference.

Here are some stories from mothers about how they created a social network for themselves:

I found online friends with similar interests. The good side of social media! I found local cloth nappy and sling library groups on Facebook, which led to finding an attachment parenting local group. After talking online for a bit I went to the meets and made some friends. I have made friends with people in national Facebook groups and we've had regional meet-ups. There is always someone there, and there's usually someone who can relate. Pocket friends. Suzanne Hancock

My husband was deployed when my youngest was three weeks old and didn't come back until she was three months old. Living on military base meant I had no family support network close by and I isolated myself so much it affected my speech when I did speak to anyone. I forced myself to go to a mum and baby yoga group and it was the best thing I did. It took me a few sessions to relax around the other mums but after that I made genuine friends I knew I could talk to. Rachael Ruddock

I went to weigh-in clinic and met another mum, our babies were one day apart and we spent the next year all surviving together. I also used the local children's centre baby groups which were a lifeline. I think for many feeling isolated and lonely and unable maybe to leave the house,

the perception of the mum who goes along to groups is that she's got it all together. But in my case it was just my way of surviving the isolation and loneliness. It wasn't about doing all the classes, it was about finding a village.
Jessica Mary Slender

My two birth experiences – and the postpartum stage – happened as an expat in two different countries. In the first the medical/birth experience was difficult and traumatic, yet the recovery and postpartum were fulfilling, happy, full of support, a tribe, a handful of mothers to guide me through and help me navigate. I was cared for mentally and physically. In the second, the birth was exactly as I wished and I was overwhelmed with care and happiness while at hospital. However, the postpartum was a lonely, cold and hard experience where I was basically dropped like a hot mess and left there to fend for myself. I had to find a tribe; care for myself and a baby. It was, in retrospect, faster to recover the first time around because of the support. Kate Brinch Sand

Choosing people to support you at home after the birth

List any supportive family members who can come into your house for a few days or weeks to look after you after your baby's birth.

When my first child was born we had an agreement with my parents that they'd come from France two weeks after the birth, once my husband had returned to work. After the birth, however, my mum couldn't wait to meet her grandson, so she asked if they could come earlier. She said that they would take care of everything in the house, the shopping, cooking, and cleaning, and that we wouldn't have to lift a finger. This proved extremely helpful in adapting to being new parents. It was wonderful to have them around during that time so we could relax and enjoy getting to know our baby without having anything else to worry about. In fact we loved it so much, that we repeated the experience after the birth of our daughter.

I would like to introduce you to the concept of having someone 'holding space' for you. I like Connor Beaton's definition of it: 'Holding space is the process of witnessing and validating someone else's emotional state while simultaneously being present to your own'. (Beaton, 2019). This means that you are truly present with someone's emotions and feelings, while being mindful of what they are saying is eliciting in you, so that you stay present and do not get dragged into your own emotions, or start talking about your own experiences. Heather Plett explains that

Holding space is not something that's exclusive to facilitators, coaches, or palliative care nurses. It is something that ALL of us can do for each other – for our partners, children, friends, neighbours, and even strangers who strike up conversations as we're riding the bus to work. (Plett, 2015)

Here is an example of how my mother held space for me when I faced the challenges of a crying baby. When my daughter was three months old my husband had to go away for work for three weeks. With a three-month-old and a three-year-old, I couldn't face being on my own for that long, so I moved to France to my parents' house for that time. Having two other adults there most of the time made looking after my children so much easier. Not only were there other people to cook, clean, and be another pair of hands to hold the baby or look after my preschooler while I fed his sister, but it also meant that I wasn't alone and had people to chat to. My daughter was prone to a long 'witching hour' phase in the evening, and would sometimes wake up in the night and cry with what seemed like digestive pain. It made a world of difference not to be on my own. Once my daughter woke up at 3am and screamed for over an hour. My mum heard her cry and woke up and came to be with me. She didn't do anything, but having her there with me meant that I could cope.

So when choosing your visitors post-birth, I cannot stress enough how important it is to ensure that whoever you get to support you is not only going to pull their weight, but is also going to make you feel supported in your parenting choices. A new mother's sense of confidence can be very fragile and the first few weeks after the birth aren't a good time to be around someone who makes you feel judged or inadequate.

The expectation that every man and his dog is welcome to visit in the first few days/weeks after the birth, errrrrmm no thanks. We had unwelcome visitors descend on us four days after my second baby was born and it was so overwhelming. I spent the majority of the visit hiding in my bedroom with my new baby, bawling my eyes out. After my third was born, the only visitors we had were my parents who helped with childcare for the eldest two while my husband, me and baby were back and forth between home and hospital for a few days. Emily Jane Gill

As a doula, I have had many complex conversations with clients about this. It is tricky, especially when family come from abroad, because there is no way to predict when the birth will happen and people's time might be limited. If your family comes too soon you might not even have given birth before they need to leave. You need to consider how you might feel labouring at home with family members around. I have known a couple to send their relatives to a B&B at the last minute when she unexpectedly went into labour at 38 weeks, and a couple who went to the husband's basement office during labour because the presence of the woman's parents in their house was slowing things down. Some clients, especially those who belong to cultures where the power dynamics between parents and children are different than in the West, have hired me for the first few weeks to support them until they feel that they have built enough confidence to face having their relatives in the house. Some clients choose to have a trial period with a family member in their house during pregnancy, to help them decide whether they want that person around immediately after the birth.

As a community midwife I was concerned how many postnatal visits left me sad at how isolated new mums felt. Many not leaving the house. So now I run a community walking group called Bumps to Buggies for my local district council. All are welcome to join us for fun, free, friendly walks. Connecting with other parents is so important; sharing, supporting, revealing experiences, knowledge and tips. Getting out of the house, walking and talking, making new friends. The conversations are enlightening, enriching, reassuring, even to me as a midwife. The walkers all consider the walks 'me-time'. Taking time to reflect, explore and discover their transition to parenthood. Find your community. After all, 'it takes a village...' Jenny Parsons

Other ways you can create a social support network

There are many national and local Facebook groups designed to connect parents. There are also a couple of apps, such as Mush or Peanut, which are designed to help mums to connect with other mums with similar-age children and organise meet-ups. You could ask your midwife or health visitor for signposts to local groups.

Organisations that can support you

- Doula UK, the association for doulas in the UK, has a doula directory at doula.org.uk
- Independent midwives offer private visits and/or postnatal support packages imuk.org.uk
- The Positive Birth Movement is a network of pregnancy and birth support groups, linked up by social media. www.positivebirthmovement.org
- Babywearing drop in and support groups: www.slingpages.co.uk
- Homestart is a local community network of trained volunteers and expert support helping families with young children through their challenging times. www.home-start.org.uk
- The NCT charity runs antenatal and postnatal classes, and local gatherings www.nct.org.uk
- The Motherside provides a support network and global community for all mums and mums-to-be, as well as local meet-ups themotherside.org
- Calmfamily provides consultations and classes to educate and support parents so that their families can have calmer relationships that optimise children's development www.calmfamily.org
- The Daisy Foundation offers antenatal and postnatal classes thedaisyfoundation.com
- Netmums www.netmums.com
- Gingerbread is a charity that supports single-parent families www.gingerbread.org.uk

Support for mental health/birth trauma
- For a list of practitioners trained in a fast birth trauma release technique called the Rewind technique, see www.traumaticbirthrecovery.com

- Make Birth Better is a collective of parents and professionals working together to end suffering from birth trauma. www.makebirthbetter.org
- Mind is a mental health charity, with a section on postnatal depression www.mind.org.uk
- Mia Scotland is a perinatal psychologist www.yourbirthright.co.uk
- The Pandas foundation for perinatal mental health www.pandasfoundation.org.uk
- SHaRON is a peer support based ehealth system, available via a mobile phone app and associated website. www.sharon.nhs.uk

Breastfeeding support

- National Breastfeeding Helpline, www.nationalbreastfeedinghelpline.org.uk. Tel: 0300 100 0212
- The Association of Breastfeeding Mothers (ABM) abm.me.uk
- The Breastfeeding Network (BfN), which includes the Drugs in Breastmilk Information Service. www.breastfeedingnetwork.org.uk
- La Leche League www.laleche.org.uk
- NCT www.nct.org.uk Tel: 0300 330 0700

Some of the charities above provide local drop-in groups too.

- Baby Cafe provides drop-in support for pregnant and breastfeeding mums www.thebabycafe.org
- Lactation Consultants of Great Britain, www.lcgb.org. The professional association for qualified lactation consultants. Members provide advice, support and consultations on breastfeeding in the UK.

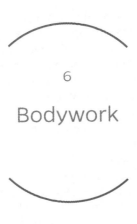

6

Bodywork

Because you and your baby are emotionally and physically vulnerable, you will be wise to follow certain guidelines. No matter where or how you had your baby, a long period of postpartum nurturing is essential. Let yourself feel like a pampered queen; you deserve to be given good care. Robin Lim

All my body has to show for it are the markings on my belly. My hip bones stayed a bit apart, my breasts are slightly saggy. But the saddest thing of it all is that we're told these marks are bad, but they're the only few reminders of this process we all have. Hollie McNish

The first time I saw a new mum being wrapped with Mexican rebozo scarves, I felt a deep longing mixed with an odd remembering, as if somehow my body knew that I needed it too. I have facilitated 'Closing the Bones' ceremonies and massages for hundreds of women, as well as training people to offer them. Every time the women taking part, whether they receive or witness the treatment, respond emotionally. When I demonstrated rebozo wrapping for a group of babywearing instructors, there was a new mother there whose baby was only three days old, so it made sense that we wrapped her. As we all held rebozo scarves wrapped tightly around her body, I read a poem, and led a simple song. When I opened my eyes after the singing, almost every woman in the circle was in tears. One of them said 'I've had nine children, and nobody has ever done anything like this for me'.

Given the tremendous changes a mother's body goes through in pregnancy and birth, it is perhaps not surprising that cultures around the world use bodywork to rebalance and restore the new mother. This is not just 'massage', but specific bodywork designed to help speed up the healing process after a mother has given birth.

When you grow and birth a baby, your whole body undergoes a remarkable transformation. Your uterus grows from the size of a pear to that of a watermelon. Your pelvis tilts forward, the curves of your spine increase and the muscles and ligaments around your belly stretch and grow. The organs inside your abdominal cavity are pushed up to accommodate the growing baby. During the birth, your uterus, pelvis, pelvic floor and vagina open and stretch to let the baby out. Then, after the baby is born, your body has to undergo all those changes in reverse, along with tremendous hormonal changes, and the beginning of lactation.

With this in mind, it seems illogical that in the West we no longer have any process in place to ensure that bones, soft tissue and organs return to an optimal position. All new mothers would benefit from some kind of 'MOT' from a postpartum manual therapist, because it is easier to prevent or treat problems as they arise, rather than letting them set into a pattern that becomes more difficult to resolve. Traditional postpartum wisdom across the world includes massage, binding and manipulations designed to help speed up healing and avoid future problems. Besides the therapeutic effect of birth-specific bodywork, any type of loving touch releases feel-good hormones like oxytocin.

Some say that birth is like running a marathon. Every athlete knows that rest and recovery are an important part of the process. I'm no marathon runner, but I was fascinated to see the similarities between marathon recovery and birth. Recommendations include recovery-specific nutrition, rehydration, pain and muscle recovery (including Epsom salt baths, for muscle soreness), massage, a period of rest, and there is even a mention of the post-exercise blues that come after a big event. (See www.theguardian.com/lifeandstyle/2018/apr/22/everything-you-need-to-know-about-recovering-from-a-marathon).

Not only do we no longer have body-nurturing practices post-birth, we also have unhealthy expectations of the postpartum body, seeing it as undesirable and ugly, and feeling immense pressure to 'lose the mummy tummy' and fit back into our jeans. This is damaging to the self-esteem and mental health of new mothers.

Midwives and doulas, in contrast, have a realistic view of the postpartum body, and we know that it takes a long time for new mothers' bodies to recover from growing and birthing a baby, and that the women who 'snap back' into shape after birth are few and far between. Luckily there are initiatives to show what real postpartum bodies look like such as www.4thtrimesterbodiesproject.com and thehonestbodyproject.com.

French medical doctor and yoga teacher Dr Bernadette de Gasquet, who specialises in birth preparation and postnatal rehabilitation, explains in her book *Mon corps après bébé* that the first six weeks is a transitional period, when everything is soft and pliable, when there is a great opportunity to heal from the birth. She recommends a programme of simple exercises to be done during this time.

When I attended Spinning Babies training a few years ago I was shocked when the trainer, a chiropractor, said it took women on average 8 to 10 *years* to seek professional help for issues like stress incontinence. As a doula I have encountered many new mums with symptoms that weren't normal, but got missed because they believed that it was to be expected, had no idea where to find professional help, or were too embarrassed to bring it up.

I supported a new mother who was suffering from double incontinence after her birth, and I accompanied her to several appointments at the local hospital. No one, despite an MRI scan, could identify what was causing the issue. After a while I suggested she might find it helpful to visit an osteopath. Her coccyx (tailbone) was not only misplaced, but also dislocated, and when treated her symptoms improved almost immediately. Some of the pelvic floor muscles attach to the coccyx, so if the coccyx isn't in an optimal position, the pelvic floor cannot function properly. In her midwifery thesis, French midwife Juliette Danis mentions this as being common:

> *The coccyx is normally mobile but it can be caused to dislocate to allow the release of the fetus. If it stays in this position, it is the source of pain, stool incontinence or constipation since the pubo-rectal muscle can no longer contract and relax normally.* (Danis, 2012)

A lack of understanding of what is normal post-birth, coupled with cultural acceptance that issues like stress incontinence, diastasis recti (separation of the abdominal muscles), and uterine or bladder prolapse are part and parcel of motherhood, contributes to the overall lack of support for new mothers.

France, as far as I know, is the only Western country that has a programme of pelvic floor re-education built into the health system. Every new mother gets offered ten free sessions of treatment, carried out by a physiotherapist or midwife, usually 6 to 8 weeks after the birth. The French health system recognises that a weakened pelvic floor can have many consequences, such as urinary leakage, risk of incontinence or organ prolapse (most commonly during the menopause). In the UK women are usually given a leaflet about pelvic floor exercises, which can help some women; however, it can be challenging to do the exercises properly. Without support, it can also be difficult for new mothers to find time to do the exercises.

Around the world, postpartum specific bodywork is (or was) part of normal care for new mothers. This often includes massage and binding with a cloth. Each culture has a slightly different approach, but the goal is to restore and 'close' the mother after the birth, and help speed up the natural healing process. These rituals usually encompass the understanding that there is a physical process that needs to be completed (helping return the body to its non-pregnant state), and an emotional/ spiritual aspect (honouring the birth process and the emotions associated with it, as well as the tremendous change to identity).

In 2013 I attended a workshop at a doula retreat called 'Closing the Bones'. This was taught by Dr Rocio Alarcon, an ethnobotanist and shaman from Ecuador who has a doctorate in Philosophy-Ethnopharmacology from University College, London. Dr Alarcon explained that if we did MRI scans on pregnant women we would see how the hips open during pregnancy, and that after birth it is paramount to help them return to their normal width, otherwise mothers suffer from pelvic instability and leak energy. She explained that in Ecuador, women would be given this massage within hours of birth, and at least five or six times during the first 40 days. The massage stimulates blood flow and moves fluids, stimulating the release of hormones and the immune system, and toning muscles and tissues. It includes rocking the pelvis with a rebozo shawl, massage of the abdomen, hips and chest/arms, and using the rebozo to wrap the pelvis.

I have been offering and teaching this process to women ever since. I have worked extensively with Cambridge osteopath Teddy Brookes to understand the effects on joints and organs, which confirmed many positive effects on spinal and pelvic joints and associated soft tissues, as well as on diastasis recti. Together we developed a new version of this massage called the Postnatal Recovery Massage, which is more extensive and is done on a massage table as opposed to a mat on the floor.

Postnatal wrapping also appears to be used worldwide. I used to think that using a girdle after birth wasn't a good idea, because my grandmother had worn a corset most of her life. Her stomach and back muscles weren't strong enough for her to be able to function without it, which made me believe that this kind of support would only cause weakness.

When I discovered that postnatal wrapping is used all over the world, I discussed it with my osteopath, who told me he could see how useful it would be as a short-term treatment. To put it simply, using a wrap around your pelvis or abdomen after birth helps support unstable joints and muscles. Rowena Hazell gave birth to triplets, and afterwards couldn't breathe properly:

As I tried to get back out of the pool, I had a weird sensation of not being able to breathe, as if all my body was suddenly too heavy. On the postnatal ward I couldn't sit up or stand for more than five minutes without finding breathing difficult. I was having to be wheeled across to NICU in a wheelchair because I couldn't walk far. The midwives didn't know why, and looked at me quite oddly when I said I needed to use a wheelchair. One of the other mums I met had brought a corset in, because she said that she had had severe diastasis recti before. The mum described it to me as your diaphragm not holding everything in, so it falls out of the bottom of your tummy. This was exactly what it felt like was happening to me! The midwives on the ward sent a physio to see me. The physio made a corset out of a double layer of their largest Tubigrip, and immediately I could breathe, sit up, and walk again with ease.

As far as I'm aware, midwife Juliette Danis's thesis is the only scientific study of postpartum binding that exists. She used a simple binding around the pelvis, applied the day after the birth for an hour. She used a set of written and visual questionnaires to evaluate its effect on pain in the pelvic area on a group of 160 women (80 receiving the wrapping and 80 controls). 64% of women described an improvement in their pelvic and perineal pain after the treatment. 79 out of 80 of the women who received the binding said they would recommend it. Danis concludes that care given to the women after birth using massages or wrapping has a positive effect both physically and psychologically, and symbolically helps to redraw the contours of the body. She believes midwives should suggest the wearing of pelvic belts for 21 days after birth as recommended by traditional societies.

This reflects my experience of giving Closing the Bones massages to new (and not so new) mothers: it is not only a pleasant massage, it is also a ritual that celebrates and honours the new mother, and can be very healing both physically and emotionally (regardless of whether the birth was a positive experience or not). Here are some testimonials from women who have had the massage:

Amazing, emotional and cleansing. I feel very supported as a new mum and feel hugged by the love this ceremony brings. Anon

It was a wonderfully relaxing experience and I felt very comforted and calm afterwards. But it was the day after I noticed the benefits even more. Prior to the massage I was getting up from sitting on the sofa or a chair with my legs wide in the same way I would as if I was pregnant. Following the massage my hips feel 'tighter' in a good way and more relaxed. I am also rising from sitting in much better alignment as before my pregnancy. Vicky

Sophie took time to explain the massage and made me feel completely at ease. She carefully arranged the room and made it feel like a cosy space with beautiful aromatherapy oils and calming music. The massage felt incredibly calming and nurturing and I felt very relaxed (almost went to sleep!) I felt a lot of tension which I was holding from the birth just disappear. Kate

The treatment gave me a space to weep and helped me heal from the labour, to start letting go of all the hurt. It allowed me to acknowledge how difficult my pregnancy was. It helped me to focus on self-care. I was able to walk better, and everything started shifting back in place. Seema Barua

Juliette Danis had one new mother undergo an MRI scan with the wrapping in place, which demonstrated that the sacro-iliac joints were decompressed and that the bladder and uterus were pulled back up (Chadelat, 2019). The wrapping also produces a reduction of the lumbar lordosis and better oxygenation (due to the diaphragm being freed), and wrapping the whole body in sequence facilitates the circulation of cerebrospinal fluid along the spine. In a Norwegian survey of therapies for pelvic joint pain, 76% of women who used a pelvic belt during or after pregnancy reported temporary improvement of symptoms (Maclennan and Maclennan, 1997).

Another advantage of wrapping the pelvis or abdomen is that it will help to keep the new mother's core warm. Warmth is important in many postpartum practices, even in hot countries, and may include wearing extra clothing and blankets, steam baths, massages and wraps with 'hot' herbs, lying above heated bricks or coal or near a fire (Dennis, 2007; Grigoriadis, 2009). New mothers may also drink hot liquids and eat hot and warming foods.

Many types of cloth can be used to wrap your pelvis or abdomen, such as scarves, rebozos, pashminas and babywearing wraps (both stretchy and woven), so you could use any of these that you already have in your home. Some women prefer to use velcro belts. The easiest and comfiest belts have a double velcro system that allows you to tighten the belt/girdle with very little effort. In the UK there are two brands that I find excellent for pelvic and/or abdominal support. For pelvic support only, during and after pregnancy, the sacroiliac pelvic belt from Belly Bands (bellybands-uk.com), or the Serola sacroiliac belt (www.serola.net) both work well. For pelvic and abdominal support, the pregnancy and caesarean 3-in-1 belly band from Belly Bands can be used in pregnancy, postpartum and post-caesarean. It is comfortable and easy to use, and the standard size fits from size 6 to 16. Like jeans, it's best to try before you buy, so you can see what works best for you.

Binding might help during pregnancy too, especially if you suffer from PGP (pelvic girdle pain). It won't treat the issue (only a manual therapist like an osteopath, chiropractor or specialist physiotherapist can do that), but it might help alleviate symptoms. The Pelvic Partnership, a charity that provides information and support for PGP states:

Support belts can be helpful to manage symptoms between treatments by keeping your pelvis supported in the correct position and helping to stabilise it. However, if you wear one without first having your pelvic joint alignment checked, it is likely to aggravate your pain. If your joints are not properly aligned, pushing them together with a belt can cause more irritation and pain at the joints. Tubigrip™ is often given out, but is difficult to put on, is often not the correct size and, again, should only be used in conjunction with treatment, so ask for more information about your options if you are just offered Tubigrip™. Often the most helpful support (once your pelvis is well aligned) is a sacroiliac support belt.

I learned about post-caesarean binding after a friend had her baby by caesarean in Bangkok and her abdomen was bound the next day in the hospital. She says she healed much better than when she had her next child in Norway, where there was no binding. A published paper on the topic found that binding post-caesarean increased mobility and reduced pain (Cheitez et al, 2010).

Interestingly, wrapping after the postpartum used to be recommended in the UK. In *An Introduction to Midwifery* (Donald, 1915) it says:

The binder should consist of a piece of stout calico, or

other strong material, about 18 inches wide and 4 feet long. When applied, the lower border should reach a hand's breadth below the widest part of the hips and should be drawn tightly and fastened securely with a safety pin or long straight pin, so that it may not work up above the hips. The middle part of the binder must be made sufficiently tight to give a sense of support, but the upper border should be rather loose as to not interfere with the patient's respiration. The binder is used merely to give external support to the loose abdominal wall.

Similarly:

It has already been observed that a bandage, wide enough to cover the whole length of the abdomen, is to be applied directly after delivery. This must be worn, gradually tightened day after day as occasion requires, until the patient is permitted to move about, when a proper and nicely adjusted belt should be substituted for it. This support will afford great comfort in all cases, but especially to those mothers that have already had many children, or a few in quick succession; (...) This belt must be worn so long as the abdominal muscles appear to require its support (Bull, 1849)

The oldest reference I found was in a book about Aristotle published in 1791:

Let the woman afterward be swathed with fine linen cloth, about a quarter of a yard, chaffing the belly before it is swathed with oil of St John's Wort; after that, raise up the matrix with a linen cloth, many times folded, then with a linen pillow or quilt, cover her flanks, and place

*the swathe somewhat above her haunches, winding it
pretty stiff* (Salmon, 1791).

Binding might have been practised more recently than this
in the UK, because midwife Siobhan Taylor told me:

*I remember my grandmother telling me that I should do
this after the twins in 1987. Everyone I mentioned it to
thought it was a crazy idea. I was even told that if your
muscles were supported, they would never regain their
former strength!*

I would like to see postnatal bodywork and massage
become the norm again. For a directory of people trained to
offer Closing the Bones or postnatal recovery massage see
closingthebonesmassage.com. If you support parents, I offer
an online course on rebozo techniques for support during
pregnancy, birth and the postpartum period at sophiemessager.
com/rebozo-online-course.

Another important aspect of postpartum bodywork is
relaxation. In addition to or instead of massage you could try
listening to music or audio tracks (there are plenty of free apps
offering guided relaxation). Learning relaxation techniques
for labour, such as breathwork and meditation, will also come
in handy during the postpartum period. Mindful Mama
author Sophie Fletcher has made a series of new motherhood
relaxation tracks available to download for free at www.
mindfulmamma.co.uk. *The Little Book of Self-Care for New
Mums* is also full of ideas to support a relaxing postpartum
(see further reading section).

An easy way to nurture your postpartum body is to have
a bath. Any frazzled new mother will benefit from a relaxing,
uninterrupted bath, especially if feel-good products have been

added to it. (If you cannot have another adult looking after your baby, bathing with your newborn can also calm you both down. Avoid the use of products in this case.) Water is used in purifying rituals around the world to mark spiritual events and life transitions, so it feels fitting that it should be used after birth too. The use of warm water and/or steam is also part of many postpartum traditions, such as steam baths, sweat lodges, saunas or vaginal steaming (Epstein and Arvigo, 2018; Dennis et al, 2007). If this appeals to you, you could make it into a ritual bath to celebrate or release emotions, with salt and/or herbs. It is more about the intention than the products. A cup of sea salt and a few sprigs of lavender would do the trick. If you cannot find the time to have a full bath, a sitz bath or a foot bath might still feel wonderfully soothing.

I like to give new mothers a simple 'teabag' to use in the bath made from healing plants such as lavender and rose. If you are going to visit a new mother, she may appreciate bath products such as herbal salts and herbs. Doula and herbalist Jo Farren offers a set of wonderful nurturing products including a healing herbal bath, bath salts and a relaxing roll-on (www.jofarren. co.uk). Neal's Yard has a new mother range too. Some mothers like to add Epsom salts (available from chemists) to their postpartum bath in order to restore tired muscles (magnesium is absorbed through the skin, and Epsom salt baths are used by some athletes for recovery).

How to get support for your body after birth

Consider bodywork treatments as an investment in your future health. Many pregnant women are happy to pay for pregnancy massage because it is 'for the baby', but feel reluctant to pay for it once the baby has been born. Yet the baby and the family as a whole will benefit immensely from the mother being nourished physically. If friends and family want to buy presents, you could ask for vouchers towards postnatal massage or visits to a manual therapist who specialises in new mothers' health, such as an osteopath, chiropractor or female health physiotherapist. There is more benefit in having repeated treatments. Some doulas trained in Closing the Bones or other postnatal massages offer packages for postnatal support that include several massage sessions.

The big advantage of postnatal bodywork is that you don't need to do the work! Someone who is skilled at working with postpartum bodies can work on your body and manipulate you in a way that will promote healing while you rest. As Jenny Allison says in *The Golden Month* 'massage is very valuable as a passive form of exercise without the mother using any of her own energy, her circulation is stimulated and she gets the pleasure and sense of wellbeing that comes with exercise.' You do not need to wait six weeks before you begin postnatal bodywork.

If you are a family member or friend of an expectant or new mother, why not buy her a voucher for a postnatal treatment? Or you could offer her a simple shoulder rub, or a hand or foot massage. You can massage shoulders through clothing, and for hands or feet olive or coconut oil from the kitchen will work just fine, though scented oil will add to the feel-good effect. You do not need to be trained in massage, just like you do not need training to give hugs. Intention is everything: if your intention is for the new mother to feel your love, that's what she'll feel.

If you're a birth worker, midwife, health professional, doula, educator or therapist, talk to your clients about the importance of getting treatment and support if they struggle with anything physical after the birth, and encourage them not to delay seeking help.

If you're a new mum, talk to your midwife, health visitor or GP about any concerns that you may have about your physical health and wellbeing after birth. There is no such thing as a stupid question. If you're worried, please ask for help. If the six-week check appointment is too short to cover everything you need, do not hesitate to ask for another appointment to discuss your concerns more specifically.

Get recommendations for a local manual therapist, such as an osteopath, chiropractor, or female pelvic health physiotherapist You might also benefit from seeing such a therapist during pregnancy, as they can work wonders to alleviate common pregnancy ailments such as PGP (pelvic girdle pain), and give your pelvis an MOT prior to birth (increasing the odds of a well-aligned baby and therefore an easier birth). After the birth it is a good idea to get checked to make sure your pelvis and abdominal soft tissues are balanced and healing well.

Some postnatal exercise classes, such as postnatal yoga and pilates, run by practitioners who have done specialist training in this area, can also be very helpful. Some of these classes include Birthlight Yoga, which have time built in for socialising too. Birthlight also has a simple postnatal recovery booklet full of safe, easy to follow and effective exercises that can be ordered from their website.

If you attend postnatal exercise classes, make sure to check the trainer's background and whether they have undergone specific postpartum training.

Dr Bernadette de Gasquet favours the use of hypopressive exercises to lift the abdominal organs and avoid pressure on the pelvic floor. Hypopressive exercises are well known in France, and considered the best form of postnatal rehabilitation available. They are still relatively new in the UK. The technique is simple: you breathe out fully, then, without taking in any air (you can pinch your nose to help) open the ribcage as if you were breathing in. Decreased pressure in the thoracic cavity draws the stomach in and the pelvic floor and uterus up. Doula and Pilates teacher Justine Sipprell offers hypopressive training for pelvic floor rehabilitation.

Plan and learn to wrap and support your pelvis and/or abdomen, whether with a piece of cloth or a velcro wrap. You could also use something as simple as a pregnancy belly band or a Haramaki (a Japanese stretchy cotton tube for your belly, which helps keep your core warm, www.nukunuku.co.uk). Having the core of your body insulated helps keep your whole body warm.

Postnatal bodywork links:

- The mummy MOT provides a listing of women's health physiotherapists who have trained to do a new mother's physical assessment www.themummymot. com
- Birthlight is a charity that provides yoga and aquanatal classes for pregnancy and new mothers, as well as baby yoga and baby swimming classes. The classes allow time for socialising. www.birthlight.com
- Carifit provide lives and online exercise classes done with a baby in a sling www.carifit.co.uk
- Dance like a Mother provides babywearing dance classes www.dancelikeamother.com. If you are looking at joining a postnatal babywearing exercise class, you might want to check that the person running the class has postnatal fitness training as well as babywearing training.

Some online postpartum diastasis/core restore rehab programmes recommended by physiotherapists:

- laurenohayon.com/offerings/restore-your-core
- onestrongmama.com
- www.holisticcorerestore.com

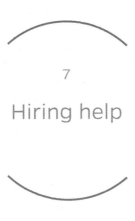

7

Hiring help

If a doula were a drug, it would be unethical not to use it.
Dr John H. Kennell

*Postpartum is a time when mothers are very conscious
of straddling the worlds of the spiritual and physical.
Doulas may help mothers integrate these worlds. With so
much occurring within her body, heart, and soul, she will
begin to realize just how intimately she is connected to all
creation. You, as her doula, can help her know that the
physical cannot be separated from the spiritual, nor the
spiritual from the physical.* Robin Lim

Alongside all the other support measures we are considering,
a doula can provide a truly unique form of support that you
might not have considered. I know this might come across as
biased, because I am a doula, but I also hired one myself so I
know how much of a difference it can make. Your doula might

be the only person around who is unbiased and whose sole goal is to make you feel confident and supported.

Some parents ask me to explain the difference between a nanny and a doula. I know there are some overlaps and that some nannies are amazingly supportive to new mums. But generally a nanny is hired to look after your baby so you don't have to, and when she leaves you might be none the wiser when it comes to babycare and mothering. Doula support might involve some babycare tasks too, and some doulas do provide overnight support. But a doula's prime focus will be you, and making sure you feel supported. A doula will also make sure that she 'works herself out of a job': she will help you work out babycare and motherhood so that by the time she leaves, you no longer need her to feel confident.

What is a doula?

A doula supports families through the pregnancy, birth and postnatal period. Often people have heard about birth doulas, but they do not know that postnatal doulas exist. Some doulas support birth, some offer support postnatally, and some do both. Doulas registered with Doula UK, the national association for doulas, have undergone an approved doula preparation course and a mentoring process with a number of clients before becoming recognised.

Doulas are lay supporters, and do not offer clinical care, but a mix of emotional, practical and informational support. A commonly used analogy is that a doula is like a Sherpa. If you were going to climb Everest, you would take your partner, but you would also hire someone to help you navigate the mountain. A doula is there to support you unconditionally without judging you or telling you what do to. Instead, a doula will help you navigate through the options available, and signpost you to information or other professionals as needed.

The work doulas do, whether for birth or postnatal support, is more about being than doing. In our culture we like to measure things, so people might ask 'What did your doula do?', but because most of the work we do is holding space and reflective listening, it might not look like we are doing much. We might look like we're just having a cup of tea with a new mother, but what we are actually doing is validating her experience and helping her make sense of it. Even parents who have had a doula find it difficult to put into words how the doula made them feel. And yet, as a wise doula once told me: anybody can do the dishes, but having a happy family eating out of those dishes is priceless.

Doula UK says:

The actual tasks in the practical support postnatal doulas provide varies enormously, and one of the big benefits of having a postnatal doula is that they are there to support the family, not carry out a specific task, so they do what is needed (within reason!). This can be help around the house, looking after baby while mum (and her partner) nap, helping with older siblings, making meals, helping with dinner time or the school run, helping overnight so the parents get more sleep... even walking dogs or wrapping Christmas presents. Whatever is needed to help a family relax and have a positive experience of life with a baby.

As well as getting to know you and providing emotional, practical and informational support, a doula can support you through the birth of your baby, which can have a very significant effect on how positive your birth experience might be. This alone can positively affect your postnatal experience. The Evidence Based Birth website reviewed the evidence on doulas using the Cochrane review (Dekker, 2019) and showed that having continuous support had the following effects:

- 25% decrease in the risk of Caesarean; the largest effect was seen with a doula (39% decrease)*
- 8% increase in the likelihood of a spontaneous vaginal birth; the largest effect was seen with a doula (15% increase)*
- 10% decrease in the use of any medications for pain relief; the type of person providing continuous support did not make a difference
- Shorter labours by 41 minutes on average; there is no data on if the type of person providing continuous support makes a difference
- 38% decrease in the baby's risk of a low five minute Apgar score; there is no data on if the type of person providing continuous support makes a difference
- 31% decrease in the risk of being dissatisfied with the birth experience; mothers' risk of being dissatisfied with the birth experience was reduced with continuous support provided by a doula or someone in their social network (family or friend), but not hospital staff

There isn't as much published evidence on postnatal doulas, but there is plenty of evidence that having postpartum support affects the experience of the new family positively, including having a protective effect on mother-baby interactions, mother-partner interactions and postpartum depression (Grigoriadis et al, 2009; Uvnäs-Moberg 2013). There is some evidence that postnatal doula support positively impacts postnatal mental health (Gjerdingen et al, 2013). Another important aspect of postnatal doula support is that doula-supported mothers are more likely to be able to breastfeed (Edwards, 2013; Stockton 2010). Not only does a harmonious breastfeeding relationship promote the release of feel-good hormones like oxytocin, which in turn helps bonding, but there is also evidence that women who wanted to breastfeed but couldn't experience grief and trauma (Brown, 2019). I am not going to go into a lot of detail here about postnatal mental health, because it's a big topic and others have written extensively about it. *Why Postnatal Depression Matters* by Mia Scotland, in this series, is a wonderful book and so is the illustrated *Good Moms have Scary Thoughts* (Kleiman, 2019).

In her book *The Hormone of Closeness*, oxytocin expert Kerstin Uvnäs-Moberg explains:

First and foremost, the doula might be supporting the woman in a purely physical way, but she is also present as emotional support. She listens to the needs of the mother and reassures her. She is compassionate and her continuous closeness creates peace and trust. She simply stimulates the mother's oxytocin release and increases her sensitivity to oxytocin by her closeness and presence.

While you could hire a doula to support you only in the postnatal period, hiring a doula that can support you through the birth *and* the postnatal period will bring you a double whammy: someone who will help you explore your options for birth, and who can help you prepare for the postnatal period in advance. Plus, by the time she turns up to support you after the birth, she will also be someone who you have come to trust and feel safe with.

Besides having a positive impact on your birth and wellbeing, a doula will also have a positive impact on your ability to rest. A doula can hold the baby while you sleep, or take a bath, or simply get a bit of much-needed baby-free time.

She's an experienced extra pair of hands around the house, and can do light household tasks such as cooking, tidying up, light cleaning, showing you how to breastfeed lying down, showing you how to co-sleep safely, showing you how to use a sling and helping you find creative ways to get as much rest as possible when she's not around. Doulas are like the fairy godmothers of perinatality. Of all the help you can have, a doula is likely to make the biggest difference to your experience.

Some other things a postnatal doula can do:

- Be a sounding board, to listen reflectively and help you make sense of your feelings and of the experience as you undergo the new mother metamorphosis, and help you see that struggling through that stage is normal and does not make you a bad mother.
- Reassure you that you are doing OK as a mother, and point out all the great loving things you are doing for your baby but cannot see yourself.
- Help you see all the amazing things you are achieving when it feels like you are doing 'nothing'.
- Help boost your confidence and reduce feelings of inadequacy, guilt and shame.
- Help reframe the normalcy of how needy and clingy tiny human infants are, and that you aren't spoiling them if you respond to your instinct to hold them.
- Encourage you to rest and prioritise your wellbeing, and help you manage priorities.
- Take care of the tasks that are important to you in your home.
- Help you get a sense of the fleeting nature of infancy, and that it won't always be this intense.
- Help keep you well fed.
- Keep you company and make you feel less isolated, as

well as helping you build a new social network.
- Help you find ways of managing your time.
- Help transform the early postpartum weeks from a difficult and uncomfortable period of growth to one of understanding and acceptance.

Here are some stories from women who had a postnatal doula:

My postnatal doula was incredible. She helped me latch the baby on, and feel calm around breastfeeding because she looked after the other two children. My husband, who has chronic fatigue, was able to rest, and he was relaxed and reassured that his wife had got help, so he was able to look after himself physically. My family was completely supported, and she was really flexible. Seema Barua

After an unexpected long induced labour and birth in the hospital, both my husband and I were physically and emotionally exhausted. Luckily I knew a postnatal doula locally who was able to come last minute to the hospital to be with me while my husband went home for a shower and rest. She brought me snacks, helped me bond with my baby and get started with breastfeeding. Gina Leung

I had twins along with a three-year-old. My doula supported my breastfeeding, cooked dinner, made sure I napped, made sure I could have a shower and always had a smile on her face. What more could you want? Emma Renshaw

Having a postnatal doula meant I could do nothing but feed my baby and rest. I stayed in bed for a week and on the couch for a week after. Our doula would sit with me

and talk through anything I was processing. She would cook food for lunch and more for the freezer. She was a breath of fresh air when my husband, myself and our preschooler all felt frazzled from the change. It meant my husband could spend time with our older daughter and she would look after me. I recovered so much quicker from birth physically and emotionally. I felt in a good place having all that support and care. Emma Hayward

I had a long, difficult birth which ended up with emergency caesarean and it was important for me to talk about the entire experience. Why it happened, did my body fail, did I fail, was motherhood born in me? Hiring a postpartum doula was also something like a treat for myself. I could just talk about myself without being embarrassed that I wanted to talk about myself first before I talked about the baby. Milena Musilová

I had the joy of a postnatal doula after the birth of my third and final child. While I was pregnant my mother was being treated for stage 4 lung cancer. Marie was heaven sent. She mothered me, she cared for me while I busied around caring for everyone else. Marie came a few times before the baby was born. She gave me space to release my fears without hurting or stressing out my surrounding family. Marie arrived as we came home from hospital. She was like an invisible blanket of warm quiet and love. She swooped in when my tears were too heavy and chatted to my other children and baby while I tried to pull it all together. She would take the kids out for small adventures without even being asked. They came back happy and light. She fed us all the most amazing food, to this day my daughter asks for Marie pasta pesto!

It took me six weeks to fully bond and find my son. Her confidence-boosting words were working, I was gathering my strength and belief in myself again. Sarah Mosier

Nothing could have prepared me for being a new mum. I was a strong and independent 33-year-old woman and didn't need anyone for anything... or so I thought!! I had a traumatic birth experience, and neither me nor my husband adjusted well to becoming new parents. I was absolutely determined to breastfeed and I was distraught when the experience didn't come naturally to me. One night I sent a fraught email to Pippa at 1am. From that moment on I was under her wing and it was such a huge relief. I so looked forward to her visits. Sometimes I took a shower or a nap, other times I just made breakfast and ate it without a baby attached to me. Above all, I credit Pippa with helping me save my breastfeeding relationship. Her compassion, acceptance and support helped me turn a disempowering, traumatic time of my life into a brand new chapter of self discovery, acceptance and confidence in myself and my abilities. Tracy Langford

One common concern is that doulas are expensive. This is actually a myth, because as doulas are on call 24/7 for up to a month for births, most of us make far less than minimum wage per hour, and doulas go above and beyond to support their clients. Regardless, especially in a system where healthcare appears free (it isn't – we pay for it with our taxes), it can feel tricky to justify the expense, and some families may simply not have the funds.

Depending on whether they are mentored or recognised, and where in the country you are based, a birth doula might cost anything from £200 to £2,000, with the average around the

£600-£1,000 mark. A postnatal doula might be from £10 to £30 an hour, with an average of £15–25 an hour. You can search for doulas who cover your area at doula.org.uk.

If you cannot afford a doula, there are other options. For vulnerable families experiencing financial hardship, Doula UK has an access fund, whereby you can get a doula for free. There are also several charitable doula programmes in different parts of the UK, which offer free support for vulnerable families. You can find a list on the Doula UK website.

It can be difficult when you do not fit the criteria for free doula support, but still cannot afford a doula. In this situation I would suggest that you reach out to local doulas and ask for help: we can be very creative! Many doulas are open to bargaining or payment in kind. Personally I've done the following: volunteer work, all sorts of payment plans, part or complete skills swaps, part or complete payments from friends and family of the client. I know doulas who have swapped their services for haircuts, plumbing work, a sofa and a holiday rental. I have swapped doula support against massages, crafts and a babywearing course.

Some doulas encourage clients to donate and/or tip towards supporting less well-off families. Once, a client I supported through her first birth rehired me for her second, but ended up moving abroad halfway through her pregnancy. She still sent me the full fee, so a mother who couldn't afford a doula could have my support instead. I used the money to support a woman who had left a difficult relationship while pregnant.

Many new mothers live far away from their family, or their family members are busy with their own lives, so it makes sense to invest in paid help if you can possibly afford it. Here are some stories from women who raised the funds for postnatal support in a creative way:

A group of internet friends paid for my doula for me for birth two after a traumatic birth. They'd known from my social account that I was in a rough way, subversively found out how much they cost, clubbed together, made up a ridiculous reason to know my PayPal account, and sent over the full whack. Meg Hill

Friends threw a party/concert, with an entrance price, openly promoting it as a fundraiser for a doula. It was a good night out and did the job! Roma Hearsey

I've done skills swap (family photos for doula support and in another instance a doula client looked after my cat for a few months while I was out of the country). Sara Benetti

You could ask friends and family to give donations towards a doula. The same goes for any paid support you might need after the birth.

Surveys show that new parents spend a lot of money on a new baby, splashing out an average of £1,600 on equipment alone, and £10,000 on the first year (Loveday, 2019; no author, 2014). The baby equipment market is awash with gadgets, and many parents feel that there is too much pressure to buy stuff for their baby. In one survey, 90% of parents admitted having overspent on baby equipment, with an average £5,567 wasted in total (Loveday, 2019).

So you could consider paring down your list of baby equipment to the basics, which isn't actually a lot: a place to sleep, some clothes and nappies, something to carry your baby in. Buying a sling and using it for the first six months, for example, could save you the need for a big pram and carrycot and you could simply buy a stroller pushchair when your baby is six months old. Or you could ask for second-hand baby items from friends and family, or buy second-hand, and redirect some of that money to spend on support after the birth.

You could make a list of the support that you would like to have after the birth, and ask friends and family to provide gifts towards that, rather than for the baby. New babies don't care about clothes and stuffed toys: what they need most are parents who feel strong enough to support them.

Other sources of paid help

Other hired helpers who might be cheaper than a doula are also worth considering, even if it is only for a short period of time while you find your feet. You could consider a mother's help, a nanny, or a cleaner.

I run a small business. I had a part-time nanny from when DS was six weeks old. Having a nanny was great as I could still breastfeed and rest, but also keep up with work duties. I didn't feel as isolated as other mums, as I still had plenty of interaction with colleagues. By the time my second arrived, the business had grown. We already knew we'd need a nanny full time from soon after the birth. She started when DD was three weeks old. Having a good nanny is wonderful. Ours also does light housework, the laundry, cooks lunch and collects our DS from school some days. It makes for a very nice life and the business continues to flourish. I'm lucky because my business allows me to work from home, so I can work and still be around for breastfeeding or if my daughter needs me. Jo Evershed

I hired a cleaner, so I could concentrate on breastfeeding. Kim Hughes

I had a nanny/housekeeper after having my third baby and then also after having my fourth for the first four weeks, seven days a week, 9am–6pm. I wish I could afford a doula but this was something I needed more intensively. I needed intense help for everything except looking after baby: looking after the other two then three children, cooking, cleaning, laundry... I needed someone to take over ALL my duties so I could just bond with baby, establish breastfeeding and concentrate on my healing. I also arranged a Closing the Bones session postpartum for my fourth baby. Hayet Hb

If I had known of anything locally, I would have had help both times! My husband worked away quite a bit, we had and have no family support, and my second child didn't sleep – I mean at all, really, for four years. When my husband was there we shared the nighttimes between us, but when he was away I really struggled. After three nights of only getting maybe three or four hours broken sleep, I would start to lose it a bit (or a lot!), so when he went away I would get a night nanny to come over every third night just so I was able to function. She was amazing, did everything exactly as we wanted without trying to impose her routines on us. She was like an angel, she would turn up at my house at bedtime, already with her pyjamas on under her coat. It was such a relief to have her, I honestly don't know how I would have coped otherwise. Lucy Atkinson

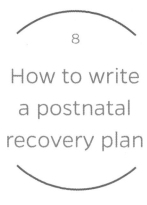

8

How to write a postnatal recovery plan

Postpartum wellness has been misinterpreted as weight loss, but in actuality, a woman's body needs careful attention for recovery and healing in the form of nourishing foods, rest, and support. Crystal Karges

Postpartum is a quest back to yourself. Alone in your body again. You will never be the same, you are stronger than you were. Amethyst Joy

Why make a postnatal recovery plan? Postnatal doula Jojo Hogan, founder of the 'slow postpartum' movement, came up with a wonderful wedding analogy:

If birth is like a wedding day (lots of planning, high expectations, being the centre of attention, lasts for about a day or so, get something special at the end), then the

postpartum should be like a honeymoon (equal amounts of planning and investment. Time, space and privacy to relax, bond and fall in love. Lots of people and services around to care for and look after you and a peaceful and blissful environment where all your needs are met for a few days or weeks).

So just like you'd plan for a honeymoon, it is well worth putting plans in place for your babymoon. Like planning for birth, it isn't about having a rigid plan. The magic isn't in the 'plan', it is in the process of exploring options and becoming informed so that you can have an experience which is as positive as possible, regardless of what happens. You can't know how you'll feel in advance, or what curveballs life might throw you, so it's worth thinking through all the possible options. That way, regardless of how your baby comes into the world, and how you end up feeling once you're home with your baby, you have at least some form of support in place.

As a birth doula, I've supported many women to write three birth plans: one for the ideal scenario, one for curveballs (for example, a change of birth place, induction of labour, instrumental birth etc), and one for a caesarean birth. I remember vividly a couple who attended my NCT classes. The baby's due date passed, and they were being pushed into consenting to induction. They hired me as a doula in early labour, and I was allowed in theatre when they had a caesarean (my local trust normally has a strict one-partner-only rule). I joined them at home then in the birth centre for many hours of labour. In the end, their baby just wasn't coming. They had been assertive about their wishes during labour, and a kind obstetrician came down from the obstetric unit to talk to them. They agreed to transfer to the delivery unit for a caesarean. As we transferred in a bit of a hurry, we weren't able to take our bags with us. Luckily, I had a copy of their birth plans in my handbag.

I pulled them out and not only did the obstetrician read their preferences and agree to support it all, but a supportive midwife also made sure the whole theatre team read their caesarean birth plan, and she negotiated for me to join them in theatre. It was a beautiful birth. The baby was placed on her chest for skin-to-skin almost immediately, and they were in a lovely bubble of oxytocin. When I met them after the birth, the mother said 'When you suggested we write a caesarean birth plan, I really didn't like it. But in the end, this meant we had a very positive birth experience, because we felt listened to and respected'.

This shows how exploring as many scenarios as possible, jotting down ideas about how you can get rest, good nutrition, bodywork and social support in place, will put you in a stronger position, regardless of what happens.

Just like when writing a birth plan, you might encounter people who dismiss your ideas. 'You can't plan birth' is a common phrase used to dismiss birth plans. Because a postnatal plan is an even newer concept, you might encounter some negativity. People might say 'You can't plan postnatal recovery', or 'You don't need that'. You might want to choose carefully who will be part of your support team, and who you discuss it with, depending on whether they are likely to be supportive or dismissive.

Another important aspect is managing visitors. This will potentially have an impact on every aspect of your recovery, for better or worse, and in particular the ability to rest, but also getting some help with chores. You might find this tricky, because in a world that glorifies busy and 'going back to normal' I've seen many new mums feel guilty at the idea of resting or refusing visits. But as a doula I have witnessed new mothers becoming exhausted by a stream of less-than-helpful visitors, as well as new parents feeling disrespected in their attempts to navigate getting to know their newborns. It can also become very complex if relatives come from abroad and move into your house if they aren't totally supportive of your choices.

The new parents' visitors from hell come unannounced very soon after the birth (sometimes even to the hospital or birth room). They bring a token present for the baby, but nothing of use for you. They expect to be waited on, and want to cuddle the baby, even if, at this early stage, you might not feel comfortable about that. They give a lot of 'well-meaning' advice about how you're doing it all wrong and undermine your already fragile sense of parenting confidence. By the time they leave, you've missed your much-needed nap, your baby is cranky from being handled by too many strangers, your house is full of crumbs and dirty mugs and plates, and you feel physically and emotionally exhausted. The new parents' visitors from heaven check what time would be convenient to visit, respect your need to have a few days to yourselves after the birth, bring you a casserole and a voucher for a postnatal massage, make you a cup of tea and a snack, only cuddle the baby if you offer that, and might send you to have a nap or a bath, and do a load of laundry or the dishes in the meantime, taking the bin out as they leave.

Warding off visitors who might not be supportive can be a challenge. Discussing your expectations ahead of time might work. If you don't want visitors but don't want to confront them, a note on the door with 'new mother and baby asleep' might do it. Another way around it is to stay in bed, or at least in your pyjamas.

We had absolutely no visitors for about a month, apart from my doula and my mum who helped with siblings and did laundry. We were gentle but very explicit with family and friends and everyone was surprisingly understanding. I'm sad it took three babies to have the confidence to put the needs of our family first. It made my recovery so much easier and the transition of a new sibling much kinder on the older children. Phyllida Warmington

Me and my husband are both Dutch so our family lives abroad. My mum was present at the birth (our wishes) and supported both me and my husband through labour. After birth she did the washing and supported me with trying to establish breastfeeding. The rest of the family came two days after my daughter was born and they respected my privacy. The in-laws gave me space and left the room when I was breastfeeding, and provided us with food and drinks throughout. My mum mainly looked after me, supported me and did anything I asked of her. Friends always asked before coming by and weren't pushy. They didn't overstay their welcome and always asked how I was doing. Healthcare visitors were really supportive and made sure I was doing okay, helped us with co-sleeping/bedsharing and I had some come by to assist with breastfeeding. My daughter was tongue tied and we had it cut privately by a midwife who again, after cutting, supported us with getting a good latch. I had a great NCT group, everyone checked in on each other at all hours of the night! Fiona Mulder

The right people – the ones who really understand what new parents need – can make a world of positive difference in your life.

As a postnatal doula, I have been hired by Dutch women for support. It isn't uncommon for Dutch women to hire postnatal doulas, because their culture is the only one I know of which has postnatal support built into the medical system, in the form of the Kraamzorg. The Kraamzorg is a cross between a postnatal doula and a maternity care assistant. She comes to the new mum's house after the birth, and helps with household tasks as well as with clinical care of the new mother and baby. Because this is part of Dutch culture, postnatal support is something that Dutch women have come to expect and they are therefore more likely to put some plans in place and hire postnatal support.

Here are the words of some women who took some steps to have a postnatal recovery plan:

Why is postnatal care important for me and how did I plan for it? Simple really... because I am making a baby inside my body. Growing, feeding and nourishing it. A little human inside me. Postnatal care is not a luxury. It's not a treat. It's a must for us and our little ones' transition into this world. I just gave birth to my third little princess five days ago. I planned my postnatal care more than any prep for my actual pregnancy and labour, so I could heal well and look after all my children and because I wanted to feel better about myself. Seema Barua

I never once thought about or planned for my recovery after the first one was born. My focus was entirely on the pregnancy and birth and what to buy for a baby. Looking back, I had gone through this incredible transformation and needed to be given time and space to just 'be'. To figure out who I was after having a baby, to let myself rest, heal, and not feel like I had to throw myself and my baby back out in to the world immediately and 'get back to my old self'. Cue a major struggle with exhaustion and postpartum depression and anxiety. I suddenly felt like simple tasks like cooking a meal became incredibly overwhelming. And having my baby in a foreign country, far from home and family, made this even harder.

I recently had my second baby, and three big differences this time were that I was back in my hometown, surrounded by family and friends who were able to support us. The second is that my husband organised a baby shower and asked everyone to bring us a meal to put in our freezer. My baby is 10 weeks now and we're still enjoying the meals that were lovingly prepared. The third reason is that I invested in my own recovery, planning to have postnatal treatments, booking to see a physiotherapist to help heal my body, and planning to seek support for my mental and emotional health. And it's given me the space I needed to slow down and be present for and committed to my transformation as a mom of one to a mom of two.

The struggle with my mental health is still there, but not nearly as bad as the first time around, and I feel so much better equipped to deal with it this time because I planned ahead and asked for help.

If you're also struggling with being a new mum, whether it's your first, or your fourth, you're not alone. And secondly, if you're pregnant, I hope this inspires you to write a postnatal recovery plan alongside your birth plan, and know that it's ok to ask for help and to be supported. Megs Lassaline

After giving birth, I stayed with my in-laws for 10 weeks. They were very helpful. They prepared all the meals for me and cooked me special 'sit-moon' food to help me recover. They helped with looking after my baby during the day so I could rest. My baby needed a lot of holding. My in-laws took turns holding my baby and rocking her to sleep. I made the decision to stay with them as I am a first-time mother and was unsure whether I could handle the stress of looking after a newborn and I'm glad I made this decision. I regained strength very quickly and my friends were amazed how quick I recovered. During the postpartum period, I received regular closing of the bone massages from Sophie, which was relaxing and refreshing. The massages helped relieve my pelvic pain and muscle ache. I highly recommend her massages. Sharon Cheung

How do you write a postnatal recovery plan?

I appreciate that I am suggesting that you write a plan for something you have no experience of and cannot predict, and that you also won't really know how you'll feel when you get there. That's okay, because regardless of how your postpartum unfolds, the basic needs of a new mother remain the same.

Remember when you write your plan that everything has the potential to have pros and cons. Just like visitors can be a blessing or a hindrance, so too can the food you choose, the way you plan to rest, your social support and so on.

Bearing in mind the four tenets of postnatal recovery: rest, food, bodywork and social support, and what is important to you, the thing to consider is how you are going to support yourself, as well as who can support you. It's a good idea to list every single idea that might help, and every single person you might be able to call on for help and support after the birth. You might find it helpful to write in the form of a spidergram or mind map rather than a list. You could use different colour pens. You could start by writing the words 'my postnatal recovery' in the middle, then the four categories above, then start writing down how you could make sure you get as much as you can from each category, as well as who could help you achieve this. There will be overlaps, but that doesn't matter. You might also find it helpful to ask mothers you know what they found most helpful. You might get some ideas you hadn't thought about, and it might help you realise what's important for you. You could also create a vision board for your postpartum, using pictures clipped from magazines.

Once you have written a draft plan, you might find it useful to enlist the help of one or two experienced mothers to review your plan. Make sure to pick supportive people! If you have a doula she will be the ideal person to help.

How long should you plan for? Because most traditional postpartum recovery practices around the world usually go on for about 30–40 days, I suggest you aim for that. But any time, however short, will be valuable, so if you can do two weeks, or even just a week, that's great: it will still make a difference to your recovery and wellbeing.

Here is a summary you can use as a prompt to write your spidergram or mind map:

Rest

- Help with household (chores, cooking, cleaning, other children etc.). Make a list of potential helpers.
- Visitors: list them/how to manage them so they do not interfere with rest. Write a 'new mother and baby sleeping' note for the door.
- Naps/sleep: when the baby sleeps/early nights/sleep with your baby
- Relaxation: techniques and apps

Food

- Batch cook and freeze
- Who could make/bring you some/meal trains
- Deliveries (supermarkets, takeaway meals, frozen, fresh, meal boxes)
- Nutritious non-perishable snacks

- Use a sling so you have your hands to fix yourself some food.

Bodywork
- Postnatal massages/Closing the Bones ceremonies
- Specialist manual therapists such as osteopaths, chiropractors, and physiotherapists
- Wrapping your pelvis/abdomen
- Keeping warm

Social support
- Friends, family, neighbours
- Hired help (doulas, nannies, cleaners...)
- Online support (social media groups, WhatsApp groups...)

Planning for the unplanned
- Navigating possible curveballs, such as if you end up giving birth by caesarean when this wasn't part of your plan and what your recovery might look like (the book *Why Caesarean Matters* has a great chapter on this), if you end up having a long hospital stay after the birth, or if your baby needs to stay in neonatal care for a while.

Gifts
- Ask people who want to give you gifts for postpartum recovery support instead.
- Make a list to suggest what you'd like: food delivery, doula or massage vouchers etc.

Mother Blessing

A wonderful way to encourage a shift in guiding your support circle towards you rather than the baby is to have a mother blessing, a mother-centred alternative to a baby shower. A circle of friends gather to honour the mother and make her feel pampered and special. Some ideas include:

- Each guest brings a bead to symbolise their good wishes for birth, and thread them into a necklace that the mother can use as a focus point during labour.
- Pass a ball of yarn around people sitting in a circle, and wrap it around one wrist, to keep on until the baby has been born.
- Giving each guest a tealight candle to light when labour starts.
- Giving the mother a hand or foot massage,
- Reading some texts or poems, sing some songs, playing some music
- Making a collage out of old magazines to represent wishes for the birth or the postpartum period.

A mother blessing is the perfect time to request gifts and pledges of support for after the birth, such as delivered meals and offers of support when you need it. Some women put up a list and ask people to tick their names against it, some people bring postpartum gifts and vouchers for the mother. It can be made even more special by bringing these people back together for a postpartum gathering celebrating the new mother a few weeks after the birth (and they can bring more gifts and food then). There is a blog about such a mother blessing, which you can find in the book link section on my website.

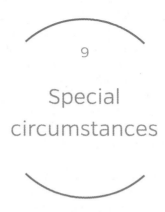

9

Special circumstances

We delight in the beauty of the butterfly, but rarely admit the changes it has gone through to achieve that beauty. Maya Angelou

How strange that the nature of life is change, yet the nature of human beings is to resist change. And how ironic that the difficult times we fear might ruin us are the very ones that can break us open and help us blossom into who we were meant to be. Elizabeth Lesser

What if you are a single mother?

The way I see it you deserve and may need even more support than someone who has a partner. It is really worth making a postnatal recovery plan and asking for help and/or hiring it if you can afford it. If you need it, Gingerbread is a charity that supports single parents www.gingerbread.org.uk.

Here are some quotes from single mums:

I was living with my mum when Ollie was born as my ex and I were still in the process of selling our house. Being with her and my stepdad was brilliant as it meant I had help with the practical adjustments I needed to make going from two kids to three. I fought against accepting their help as I stubbornly believed I should have been able to do it all on my own, but looking back I'm so grateful they were there to give me a few weeks to learn how to parent three kids before I moved into my own place and did it solo. Tara Bungard

I planned to spend the first few weeks/months in bed if that's what I wanted to do and that made all the difference. Not having any other responsibilities to fulfil made being a solo mum amazing. I had a wonderful first year compared to a lot of my friends who had to also consider their partner's needs during that time which was more stressful in many ways. A doula helped. Having my mum on hand to do cooking and washing was great. Anonymous

When I decided to have my second child I knew that I was going to do it mostly on my own. I had someone in the house where I gave birth for three days. The following week, I had various friends coming and going to bring some support. As a fiercely independent woman, I found it so incredibly hard to accept to lean onto others. My saviour was definitely slings and acceptance that my priorities were bonding and resting while trying to look after a four-year-old. Five years on, I am astonished how I managed to function while my body recovered. I would definitely choose to do things differently if I had another child. I would get more hands-on support, get more support from alignment therapists for myself and my baby, try and organise a post-partum doula, or get my mum to stay for a month or three! Lorette Michallon

I wish I had had the means to do this. I had a birth doula and used hypnobirthing which really empowered the birth. I really struggled financially, practically (none of my peers had had children at that point and I was clueless) and emotionally. I lost my friends as they didn't understand babies. For the first month I didn't have internet or TV, my doula sent me links to articles but I didn't have internet to access them on. Eventually I moved to a self-contained room at my parents' house for a year. What kept me sane was meeting other mothers at baby groups and training in babywearing and hypnobirthing – although this was also a big conflict/challenge with lack of childcare so took much longer than if there had been another parent involved, it also cost my savings and didn't make profit in the years I was single parenting. The support that would have helped was: food prep, social contact, knowing other single parents, someone to hold my baby while I washed/did household tasks, someone to say 'It's ok to balance your needs with your baby's needs'. I tried to show bravado 'I can do it' by doing things I knew would be hard such as attending festivals, travelling long distances to meet friends... I wouldn't do this again in the same situation. Anonymous

I (stupidly) had absolutely nothing in place. When my little guy was a week old and I had mastitis I called my mum in tears and she came to get me. We stayed with her for the next six weeks. I wish I had put more in place before he was born. I wish I had been able to afford a postnatal doula actually! Emma Crossley

What if your baby has to spend time in NICU? What if you have to spend longer than expected in hospital?

When I have supported parents who had to stay in hospital for a while, or when their baby needed to stay in NICU, the majority of people have asked me to delay the support they had hired me for until they were home. I understand why they chose to do this: after all, when you are in hospital, there are medical staff looking after you, so it can be easy to think that you do not need support. However, in my experience long stays in hospitals are rarely relaxing. If you're staying on the postnatal ward, you are likely to be in a bay of several beds, surrounded by other women and babies as well as visitors. It is likely that there is a medical protocol going on (such as antibiotics administered intravenously for you or your baby), which entails regular visits from midwives and/or doctors. Similarly, if your baby is in NICU the care routine can take up all of your day. In either of these situations, it is easy to get so busy with the hospital routine that you forget to look after yourself, don't eat well, and don't get any rest during the day. Tommy's, the baby loss charity, says:

If your baby is born early or poorly it can be a huge shock and you may feel that you're being asked to make big decisions while you're in a daze. You may find it hard to bond with your baby if you are frightened about whether he or she will be OK. You can be more prepared for what happens if a baby needs to go into the hospital's special care unit by reading about premature birth.

Here is what some mothers have to say:

When I had my second baby in hospital he had to stay in NICU. The hospital tried to keep me in hospital with him, but in the end I was just moving from one ward to another. My other half was staying with a friend with our oldest boy and so it was hard for us to spend time together. We were waiting for there to be space in the family accommodation but at one point I was put in this bedsit in a tower block a good 10 minute walk across the hospital grounds, I remember just bursting into tears at how horrid it was stuck away from everyone. I couldn't sit down very well because of the pain of the episiotomy so couldn't sit while visiting my son. I remember walking, walking from room, to NICU to pumping room to vending machine, it was so exhausting. In hindsight it might have been better to have stayed with the friend as well but I was in no state to rationalise anything. Rosie Dhoopun

It's day ten. We have moved from NICU to SCBU. I haven't slept more than three hours a day since I had my emergency C-section and lost 2.3 litres of blood. Just as I welcome sleep, they roll my son in. Now I must look after him. I'm delirious with exhaustion. I feel really strongly there's a need for doulas in NICU and SCBU situations. My husband was with my older child, I had been 'discharged' but was living on SCBU in a side room. There wasn't anyone looking after me at all. Zelle Baggaley

The first week in a NICU can be pretty soul-destroying. You are watching your baby strapped to wires with machines beeping all around and it's filled with a lot of tears, fear and uncertainty. From the start of week two you are pretty much running on no food and lots of adrenaline from the determination to get your baby home safe and as soon as possible. You don't eat properly, drink properly, rest, or take any care of yourself at all. The nurses are one of a kind and will listen to all your fears and questions and try their best to help you as well as giving round the clock care to your little one. However, aside from the conversations you squeeze in between rounds there is very little support for both parents during this time. Several times I could see my husband at breaking point and when I reached out the unit was told there used to be counsellors on the ward for parents, but these were taken away due to budget cuts. One thing I wished we had more than anything was support on the ward. Someone you could ask questions to, generally vent and to help us take care of ourselves. It is hard. There are no two ways about it. But if you have a good support network it will help a lot more then you realise. Katie Fountain

Support from family and other care-givers: a doula is vital when you have babies in the NICU. The strain and stresses you are under are enormous and every bit of help is needed. Just knowing that my mother-in-law would drive me in and pick me up every day was such a huge pressure taken off me and my partner who was still working and dropping off and picking up our eldest from nursery. Just having my doula to message and talk things over was amazing. Claire Walker

It is unlikely that you will have time to prepare if a long hospital or NICU stay happens, so I would like to suggest that you plan for it just in case. The same basic principles apply: how will you make sure you get enough rest (help from supportive people, such as tag-teaming with your partner and family members can be very helpful), getting nutritious food (hospital food isn't always the best, so if you can get home-cooked food delivered to you by friends and family it might make a world of difference), wrapping your pelvis/abdomen, especially post-caesarean as this may help you move more easily, and kind, listening ears to help you process your emotions.

When a woman (...) sees her baby in the NICU, she may blame herself and the choices she made. The partner and birth team can help by providing context and letting the nurses and doctors know the mother's emotional state (...). Understanding that a NICU stay is extraordinarily difficult for parents, the family can request that the hospital provides a patient advocate so they feel they have extra support in hospital. Midwives and doulas can help the family ask for their right to know what criteria the baby needs to meet before discharge is granted. (Jarecki and Mednick, 2015).

What if your baby dies

If we do not suffer a loss all the way to the end, it will wait for us. It won't just dissipate and disappear. Rather, it will fester, and we will experience its sorrow later, in stranger forms. Elizabeth Lesser

Grief is not a disorder, a disease or sign of weakness. It is an emotional, physical and spiritual necessity, the price you pay for love. The only cure for grief is to grieve. Earl Grollman

I wanted to write something about the loss of a baby because it is a subject close to my heart. I am the older sister of a stillborn baby, and I also had four miscarriages. There is still so much taboo around baby loss and pregnancy loss. What I want to say to you is this: if you experience a loss, regardless of what stage of your pregnancy you are at, you will be postpartum. You will need to grieve, and you deserve the same support as a mother who has given birth to a live baby. In fact you will probably need it more.

The tricky part is that it is likely that you will have no time to plan. I hope you can still use some of the suggestions made in this book to help you. If you are a family member or friend of someone who has experienced a loss, use this book to support them.

If you lost your baby earlier in pregnancy you might feel that your loss isn't valid. But you cannot measure grief by what it looks on paper. Your grief can be as real if your baby died when you just found out you were pregnant, or if your baby died when he was several months old. So I want to share my stories, and those of others, and I hope it helps demonstrate the need for support.

When I was eight years old my little brother, Julien, was stillborn. This was in the late 1970s, and in those days people thought that brushing things under the carpet was the right thing to do. None of us were allowed to grieve or process our feelings. There was no funeral, there was no memory box, no pictures, no footprints. I never got to see my brother and neither did my mother. We didn't talk about it, and we didn't share our sadness. But the grief was there, nevertheless. So I was left with all those unprocessed feelings, and my mind chose to forget them to protect me. I have a big blank in my memory. I can't remember my mum being pregnant, or anything after the birth. There is a part of my childhood I simply cannot reclaim because we weren't allowed to grieve at the time.

When I studied how children grieve as part of my antenatal

education diploma, I revisited this situation and had some lovely healing conversations with my mother about it. It also led me to close the circle by giving my mum a Closing the Bones massage. She was scared in case all the bad feelings came flooding back, but it was gentle and beautiful and honouring, nurturing and healing for both of us.

I also experienced four miscarriages. I started to try and conceive when I was 33. After over a year of trying and no pregnancy, we were fast-tracked for fertility tests, due to my age and irregular cycles. Everything was normal but my cycles were very long and they wanted to give me drugs to induce ovulation. I wasn't keen, so I investigated other options instead, and after three months of acupuncture, I fell pregnant for the first time.

I can still feel the raw, amazing joy I felt when the test was positive. I can still picture myself, alone in the bathroom. I looked at myself in the mirror, and I burst into tears of joy. I kept my little secret all day and then surprised my husband with the wrapped positive test in the evening. For three months I walked around in a constant state of bliss. Yes I was tired and nauseous at times, but mostly I was on a joyful high.

At 12 weeks we went for our first scan. We were very excited. Then the sonographer told us there was no heartbeat. She tried scanning me again. I was in denial, still hopeful that somehow, there had been a mistake, and that my baby would still be alive. But my baby had died.

What ensued was disbelief, numbness and shock, followed by the deepest grief I had ever experienced. I cried like I had never cried before in my life. Big, heavy, howling sobs. My arms literally ached for my baby.

This wasn't helped by my lack of understanding of my own feelings, by the lack of acknowledgement our culture gives to women who miscarry, by the lack of support, or by the inappropriate, well-meaning comments of friends and relatives who didn't know how to support a mother's grief.

- 'It wasn't a real baby' (to me it was)
- 'There was probably something wrong with it' (maybe, but this was implying I was wrong to grieve)
- 'You can have another one' (I wanted this one)
- 'At least you can get pregnant' (more grief dismissal)

Thankfully someone put me in touch with the Miscarriage Association. I rang a lovely local volunteer, Janet Sackman. She was the first person to put soothing, acknowledging words on my grief, and I still remember how important this was in the healing process. I ended up attending Miscarriage Association meetings for a while. It helped me a lot with processing my feelings and having a safe space where I could speak them without feeling judged.

But nothing was done to help heal my body, my spirit, my soul, in a holistic way. I also carried the grief and fear with me – nobody helped with that. I never experienced that feeling of bliss in any of my subsequent pregnancies (I went on to have three more miscarriages as well as two live children), because I was so scared that I was going to lose my baby again, that I didn't dare let myself be happy in a silly bid to protect myself from grief. (I have since learnt that, while common, this technique doesn't work: if you try and protect yourself by anxiously worrying about the worst possible scenario, it doesn't stop you from experiencing grief if it happens – it only robs you of joy).

When I learnt to offer the Closing the Bones massage, it made sense to me that I would offer it to women after loss, and I have seen how helpful it is. This is what some of those women said:

I came along to the Closing the Bones training about a year after my baby had died. Towards the end of the ceremony, as I was being rocked, deep shudders started going through my body and as the rebozo was pulled tight around my pelvis I felt a huge emotion that even now I am not sure what to call it. It felt as though the protective bubble I had formed around myself moved away and with that my baby – as if I was releasing him. Sobs racked my body, all the grief, the anger, the exhaustion all the disbelief of what had happened came pouring out. I hadn't realised how much I was holding on to. I felt the women form a circle around me and felt what it was like to have a safe space held for me, allowing me to just be there in my wild tumult of emotion. I heard someone singing the most beautiful song and someone stroking my hair, hands touching me sending love and support. Rosie

I have had three different losses. All the years up to having children when I felt sad I realised I had empty arm syndrome. It was a deep sadness that as I was so young was not felt I had the luxury of acknowledging. When I felt pregnant, I never fully bonded – just in case. I always felt doomed. After two more children in quick succession I learnt Closing the Bones and was lucky enough to be the subject for the full closing ceremony at the end. I could see golden light all around and I felt deeply relaxed and to have so many women touch me was a unique honour. When I got home I felt a far deeper connection to my children than I had before. Allison

Having the Closing the Bones massage helped me to accept my baby's loss and start to move forward and also forgive my body and let go of all the negative feelings. Claire

And these women, who didn't have Closing the Bones massage, but have since learned about it, feel that it would have been beneficial:

I had a miscarriage at nine weeks. I think Closing the Bones would have helped me in so many ways, but mostly emotionally, being able to share it with another woman who understands or at least who can empathise and perhaps sympathise. Who could normalise it (I knew it was common, but it would still have been nice to be told again, several times!). A healing time with another woman. That's what I would have liked. Saveria

I didn't know about Closing the Bones until recently and had not really considered it with regards to my loss, but your post made me reflect and actually had (has!) me in tears thinking about how, at the time, a 'ceremony' would have helped me so very much. I would have found a Closing the Bones ceremony beautiful in that situation, a celebration of my child, me as her mother, and a way of celebrating her life, however short it was. I would have found it healing and it would have allowed me the focus I so desperately needed to just be alone with her, and my thoughts, and my pain! Jo

If you experience baby loss, I would like to invite you to treat yourself in the same manner as a new mother would be treated if her baby was alive. The same tenets of support apply: rest, food, bodywork and social support. Try and get some time off work to recover physically, eat warm nourishing food, wrap your abdomen/pelvis and maybe get a massage when you're ready, and make sure there are supportive people and maybe therapists you can talk to.

- This article talks about the physical recovery, and what you might be missing on, after a stillbirth stillstandingmag.com/2018/08/04/postpartum-recovery-baby-loss
- Do reach out for support from a community of people which understands what you've been through, such as the Miscarriage Association (www.miscarriageassociation.org.uk)
- Sands www.sands.org.uk and Tommy's www.tommys.org are UK baby loss charities.
- Maisie Hill is a doula and traditional Chinese practitioner, and her article 'How to recover from a miscarriage' (www.maisiehill.com/blog/how-to-recover-from-a-miscarriage) has a lot of wisdom to offer:

We often believe that healing is a linear process, one in which we gradually get better, until one day, we're fine. But it's messier than that, it can be two steps forward, five steps back. You may feel like you're doing well, and then a whole new set of emotions enters your being, and with that, the possibility of having to find new ways to understand and work through them. Loved ones and colleagues may also assume that you're doing well, and be taken aback by sudden changes in mood and wellbeing. It isn't fun but it *is* healthy, and as a friend of mine says, you're exactly where you need to be. (Hill, 2019)

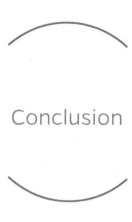

Conclusion

The vast majority of postpartum women do not need professional care. They need meals cooked for them. They need volunteer babysitters if they have other children. They need help with housekeeping. They need juices and herbal teas served to them. They need reassurance and love. Any neighbour, relative, or friend, can do these things. Yet for too many modern women, postpartum is a lonely time. If friends and family do not care for new mothers, they experience social isolation. Robin Lim

The changes taking place for both mother and baby are not only physical, they are spiritual and social. In most cultures the weeks immediately following birth are a time of protection, hedged around with specific dietary and other rules which require the active cooperation of the various women in the family and neighbourhood. Sheila Kitzinger

When I decided to write this book, my vision was to help transform our culture from one that doesn't support new mothers to one that does. I wanted to help spread the knowledge I had acquired about what postpartum used to look like, and still looks like, in cultures that have understood how important it is. I wanted to try and help shift the mindset of people who mistakenly think that the sooner a mother 'goes back to normal' the better.

What blew my mind when I was doing the research for this book was just how incredibly similar and ubiquitous postpartum practices are around the world. And while I suspected the Western world once had such practices too, I didn't expect to find written evidence of them, nor that they would be relatively recent. I share Naomi Kemeny's hope that

> *the positive effects of good postnatal care ripple outwards: anyone receiving your gift of care will know how good it feels and hopefully, in time, they will be able to provide the same support for their own friends, family and future grandchildren.* (Kemeny, 2014).

If enough new mothers experience the transformative effect of support after birth, maybe it will become normal for our society again.

What if we nurtured new mothers? I believe that, beyond the immediate wellbeing of the new mother and her partner, and her baby, there is the power to change society as a whole. Nurtured new mothers are likely to be more nurturing towards their babies, simply because while mothers are incredibly resilient, you cannot pour from an empty cup.

Because of the positive impact on society, I believe that investing in new mothers is a long-term cost-saving exercise. I have a series of hopes about what this book might help achieve:

- I hope reading about what other cultures have and what we used to have helped you understand why postpartum support is a necessity and not a luxury.
- I hope that reading about what used to happen in the UK helped you understand that this isn't an 'exotic' idea.
- I hope that reading about our culture helped you understand why what we currently have is not just abnormal; it is also detrimental to new families and society as a whole.
- I hope that have made a clear case for why rest, food, bodywork and social support are so important, and shown how we can implement them within our Western culture.
- I hope that I have provided enough examples and options for you to be able to visualise what a supportive postpartum might look like for you, design your own plan, and put it into practice.
- I hope I might have helped change the minds of a few people, not just new parents and their supporters, but anybody who might be in a position to help support new mothers.
- If you have just finished reading this book and you are an expectant or new parent, I hope that you have found ideas to help you have an easier, more supported experience after your baby is born.
- If you are a friend, or a family member of an expectant or new mother, I hope that you have found new ways to offer them support them after the birth.
- If you are a birthworker, a doula, a midwife, a health professional, an educator, antenatal or postnatal course facilitator, a therapist, or anybody who works with and supports families during the antenatal, birth

or postnatal period, I hope that this book has helped provide a framework to encourage your clients to think and plan for the postnatal period, and that it will help add useful ideas to your practice.

At the time of writing, in the midst of the 2020 COVID-19 pandemic lockdown, oddly change seems more possible than ever. Over the last week I have done shopping and provided food for vulnerable neighbours, delivered soup to a sick friend's doorstep, and exchanged missing ingredients with someone in my street. I have seen support groups being set up across the country. I hope reclaiming postpartum nurturing can ride the wave of this new-found community support.

I started this book with a paragraph comparing what a new mother's life might look like in a supportive society compared to a non-supportive one. I would like to end with what I think it might look like if we fuse traditional postpartum wisdom and our modern lifestyle in today's world:

A baby is born. The new mother knows that the community will rally round to support her. While she was pregnant she had a party to celebrate her pregnancy. She received gifts for herself, as well as pledges of support for after the birth. Friends and family respect her need for rest and schedule their visits accordingly. A neighbour organises a meal train, and people leave casseroles on her doorstep. When people visit, they lavish attention on her and praise her for how well she is doing. They offer to hold the baby while she naps and look after the household. She gets plenty of rest. She receives some postpartum specific massages or manipulations, and she wraps her belly. There are enough people around her to support her if she needs it with feeding and babycare, in ways that respect her autonomy. She is firmly in the driving seat of her recovery, and these people respect her needs, providing care without it being overwhelming. By the time a month has passed, she feels rested and competent in caring for her baby.

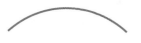

Further reading

Postpartum wisdom

Ou, H. *The first forty days, the essential art of nourishing the new mother,* Stewart, Tabori and Chang, 2016.

Allison, J. *The Golden Month*, Beatnik Publishing, 2015.

Hands, B. and Stickland, A. *Little Book of Self-Care for New Mums,* Vermillion, 2018.

McConville, B. *On becoming a mother. Welcoming your new baby and your new life with wisdom from around the world,* Oneworld, 2014.

Johnson, K.A. *The fourth trimester, a postpartum guide to healing your body, balancing your emotions and restoring your vitality.* Shambhala, 2017.

Doulas and support

Kemeny, N. *Nurturing New Families*, Pinter & Martin, 2014.

McMahon, M. *Why Doulas Matter*, Pinter & Martin, 2015.

Stockton, A. *Gentle birth companions, doulas serving humanity,* McCubbington Press, 2010.

Lim, R. *Eat Pray Doula*, Half Angel Press, 2012.

Birth

Hill, M. *The Positive Birth Book*, Pinter & Martin, 2017.

Hill, M. *Give Birth Like a Feminist*, HQ, 2019.

Brown, A. *Informed is Best: How to spot fake news about your pregnancy, birth and baby,* Pinter & Martin, 2019.

Meddings, N. *Why Home Birth Matters,* Pinter & Martin, 2018.

Schiller, R. *Why Human Rights in Childbirth Matter,* Pinter & Martin, 2016.

Hazard, L. *The Father's Home Birth Handbook,* Pinter & Martin, 2010.

Goggin, C. *Why Caesarean Matters,* Pinter & Martin, 2018.

Reed, R. *Why Induction Matters,* Pinter & Martin, 2018.

Mental health

Kleiman, K. *Good moms have scary thoughts,* Familius, 2019.

Scotland, M. *Why Postnatal Depression Matters,* Pinter & Martin, 2015.

Brown, A. *Why Breastfeeding Grief and Trauma Matter*, Pinter & Martin, 2019.

Breastfeeding

Brown, A. *The Positive Breastfeeding Book*, Pinter & Martin, 2018.

Newman, J. *Dr Jack Newman's Guide to Breastfeeding,* Pinter & Martin, 2014.

Gonzales, C. *Breastfeeding Made Easy,* Pinter & Martin, 2016.

Relationships

Taylor, E. *Becoming Us: 8 steps to grow families that thrive,* Three Turtles Press, 2011.

Fisher, D. *Baby's here! Who does what?* Grandma's Stories Ltd, 2010.

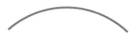

Acknowledgements

I am grateful to my parents Michelle and Jacques for being staunch supporters of my work and personal development, especially through my professional conversion from a prestigious career in science to becoming a self-employed birth worker. Maman, papa, merci. Je vous aime.

To my husband Chi, with you I feel loved, safe and supported to be exactly who I am. We have two gorgeous children and I am full of gratitude for you and our journey together. To my children, Sebastien and Charlotte, you stretched my brain and my heart into someone completely new. You are amazingly kind and empathic human beings and I am incredibly proud of you and who you are becoming.

I am grateful to Maddie Mc Mahon for being my birth doula and introducing me to the world of doulaing, and to Dr Rocio Alarcon who introduced me to the Closing the Bones postnatal massage that has influenced this book.

To the amazing group of birth worker friends who helped shape the outline and first few chapters of this book: Allison,

Alex, Attila, Azeeta, Becki, Caro, Carly, Claire, Elle, Grace, Hazel, Hilary, Japjeet, Julia, Laura, Lorette, Lynsey, Melanie, Melissa, Molly, Naomi, Nicola, Rebecca, Roma, Rosie D, Rosie K, and Wibke. Thank you for holding my hand, boosting me up and giving me feedback, and for sharing your stories!

I am grateful to all of my doula clients and the women who agreed to share their stories for this book. As Brené Brown says, 'stories are like data with a soul'. Thank you for giving this book more soul. Thank you to mothers Elle Fleming and Johanna Riha who gave me feedback on the first draft of this book.

Thanks to midwives Becky Reed and Siobhan Taylor, who reviewed the first draft as well as providing amazing anecdotes.

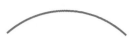

References

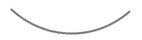

Allison, J. *The Golden Month*, Beatnik Publishing, 2015.

Badr, B.H., Jaclene, A., Zauszniewski, J.A. 'Meta-analysis of the predictive factors of postpartum fatigue'. *Applied Nursing Research*, 2017

Beaton, C. *WTF Is Holding Space. (A Man's Guide).* 2019 [ONLINE] available from connorbeaton.com/wtf-holding-space-mans-guide

Bonyata, L. 'Oatmeal for increasing milk supply'. 2017 [ONLINE] available from kellymom.com/bf/got-milk/supply-worries/oatmeal/.

Brown, A. *Why Breastfeeding Grief and Trauma Matters,* Pinter & Martin, 2019.

Brown, B. *Daring Greatly: How the Courage to Be Vulnerable Transforms the Way We Live, Love, Parent, and Lead,* Penguin Life, 2015.

Bull, T. *Hints to Mothers on the Management of Health During the Period of Pregnancy, and in the Lying-in Room,* Longman & Company, 1849.

Byrom, S., Edwards, G. and Bick, D. *Essential Midwifery Practice, Postnatal Care,* Wiley Blackwell, 2010.

Cameron, A.M. 'From ritual to regulation? The development of midwifery in Glasgow and the West of Scotland, c.1740-1840', PhD thesis, 2003.

Centola, D., Becker, J., Brackbill, D., Baronchelli, A. 'Experimental evidence for tipping points in social convention', *Science*, 2018.

Chadelat, C. and Mahe-Poulin, M. *Le mois d'or. Bien vivre le premier mois apres l'accouchement,* Presses du Chatelet, 2019.

Cheifetz, O., Lucy, S.D., Overend, T.J., Crowe, J. 'The effect of abdominal support on functional outcomes in patients following major abdominal surgery: a randomized controlled trial', *Physiotherapy Canada*, 2010.

Cleveland, L., Hill, C.M., Pulse, W.S., DiCioccio, H.C., Field, T., White-Traut, R. 'Systematic Review of Skin-to-Skin Care for Full-Term, Healthy Newborns', *J Obstet Gynecol Neonatal Nurs*, 2017.

Danis, J. 'Le serrage de bassin en postpartum', midwifery thesis, France, 2012.

De Gasquet, B. *Mon corps après bébé, tout ce joue avant 6 semaines*, Marabout, 2012.

Dekker, R. 'Evidence on: Doulas', 2019. [ONLINE] available from evidencebasedbirth.com/the-evidence-for-doulas/2019

Dennis, C.L., Fung, K., Grigoriadis, S., Robinson, G.E., Romans, S., Ross, L. 'Traditional postpartum practices and rituals: a qualitative systematic review', *Womens Health*, 2007.

Ding, G., Tian, Y., Jing Yu, J., Vinturache, A. 'Cultural Postpartum Practices of "Doing the Month" in China'. Perspectives in Public Health, 2018

Donald, A. *An introduction to midwifery. A handbook for medical students and midwives,* Charles Griffin and Co. Ltd, 1915.

Edwards, R.C., Thullen, M.J., Korfmacher, J. , Lantos, J.D. , Henson, L.G, Hans, S.L. 'Breastfeeding and Complementary Food: Randomized Trial of Community Doula Home Visiting'. Pediatrics 2013

Epstein, N. and Arvigo, R. *Spiritual Bathing,* Echo Points books and media, 2018.

Esposito, G., Yoshida, S., Ohnishi, R., Tsuneoka, Y., Rostagno Mdel, C., Yokota, S., Okabe, S., Kamiya, K., Hoshino, M., Shimizu, M., Venuti, P., Kikusui, T., Kato, T., Kuroda, K.O. 'Infant calming responses during maternal carrying in humans and mice', *Curr Biol,* 2013.

Fisher, D. *Baby's here! Who does what?* Grandma's Stories Ltd, 2010.

Gerhardt, S. *Why Love Matters: How Affection Shapes a Baby's Brain*, Routledge, 2004.

Gjerdingen, D.K., McGovern, P., Pratt, R., Johnson, L., Crow, S. 'Postpartum doula and peer telephone support for postpartum depression: a pilot randomized controlled trial', *Journal of Primary Care Community Health*, 2013.

Goggin, C. *Why Caesarean Matters*, Pinter & Martin, 2018

Goodman, J.M., Guendelman, S., Kjerulff, K.H. 'Antenatal Maternity Leave and Childbirth Using the First Baby Study: A Propensity Score Analysis', *Women's Health Issues*, 2017.

Grigoriadis, S., Erlick Robinson, G., Fung, K., Ross, L.E., Chee, C.Y., Dennis, C.L., Romans, S. 'Traditional postpartum practices and rituals: clinical implications', *La Revue Canadienne de Psychiatrie,* 2009.

Guendelman, S., Pearl, M., Graham, S., Hubbard, A., Hosang, N.,

Kharrazi, M. 'Maternity leave in the ninth month of pregnancy and birth outcomes among working women', *Women's Health Issues*, 2009.

Hammer, A., Halla, M., Scheeweis, N. 'The Effect of Prenatal Maternity Leave on Short and Long-term Child Outcomes', *Journal of Health Economics*, 2020

Henrich, J., Heine, S.J., Norenzayan, A. 'The weirdest people in the world?' *Behavioural and Brain Sciences*, 2010.

Hill, M. 'A healthy baby is not ALL that matters', 2015 [ONLINE] available from www.positivebirthmovement.org/eregrgrtg/

Hill, M. 'How to recover from a miscarriage', 2019 [ONLINE] available from www.maisiehill.com/blog/how-to-recover-from-a-miscarriage

Hsieh, C.H., Chen, C.L., Han, T.J., Lin, P.J., Chiu, H.C. 'Factors Influencing Postpartum Fatigue in Vaginal-Birth Women: Testing a Path Model', *Journal of Nursing Research*, 2018.

Huang, Y.C., Mathers, N.J. 'A comparative study of traditional postpartum practices and rituals in the UK and Taiwan', *Diversity in Health and Care*, 2010.

Hunziker, U.A., Barr, R.G. 'Increased carrying reduces infant crying: a randomized controlled trial', *Pediatrics*, 1986.

Jarecki, C.K. and Mednick, L.P. *Homebirth Cesarean: Stories and Support for Families and Healthcare Providers*, Incisio Press, 2015.

Kemeny, N. *Nurturing New Families: a guide to supporting parents and their newborn babies,* Pinter & Martin, 2014.

Kim, P., Swain, J.E. 'Sad dads: paternal postpartum depression', *Psychiatry*, 2007.

Kleiman, K. *Good moms have scary thoughts,* Familius, 2019.

Knowles, R. *Why Babywearing Matters*, Pinter & Martin, 2016.

Kurth, E., Spichiger, E., Stutz, E., Biedermann, J., Hosli, I. and Holly, P., Kennedy, H. 'Crying babies, tired mothers – challenges of the postnatal hospital stay: an interpretive phenomenological study', *BMC Pregnancy Childbirth*, 2010.

La Leche League International, *Sweet Sleep: Nighttime and Naptime Strategies for the Breastfeeding Family*, Pinter & Martin, 2014.

Lim, R. *After the Baby's Birth: A Woman's Way to Wellness – A Complete Guide for Postpartum Women,* Celestial Arts, 2001.

Lim, R. *Eat Pray Doula,* Half Angel Press, 2012.

Loveday, 'A UK Study Reveals How Much First-Time Parents are Spending on Baby Gear', 2019 [ONLINE] available from ergobaby.co.uk/blog/uk-study-reveals-how-much-first-time-parents-are-spending-on-baby-gear/

Hansford, L. 'What's The Big Deal With Skin-To-Skin?' no date [ONLINE] available from www.laleche.org.uk/whats-big-deal-skin-skin

Maclennan, A.H. and Maclennan, S.C. 'Symptom-giving pelvic girdle relaxation of pregnancy, postnatal pelvic joint syndrome and developmental dysplasia of the hip', *Acta Obstetricia et Gynecologica Scandinavica*, 1997

Marks, L. (1996) *Metropolitan Maternity: maternal and infant welfare services in early twentieth-century* London. Rodopi B.V.i. 1996.

McKenna, J. 'How Parents Can Benefit from Cosleeping', excerpt from *Sleeping With Your Baby: A Parent's Guide To Cosleeping,* Platypus Press, 2007. [ONLINE] available from www.naturalchild.org/articles/james_mckenna/parents_benefit_cosleeping.html

McKay, A. *The Birth House*, Harper Perennial, 2010.

McMahon, M. *Why Doulas Matter*, Pinter & Martin, 2015.

Negron, R., Martin, A., Almog, M., Balbierz, A., Howell, E.A. 'Social support during the postpartum period: Mothers' views on needs, expectations, and mobilization of support', *Matern Child Health J,* 2013.

No author. 2014 UK: 'First-time parents spend £492 million preparing for baby' [ONLINE] available from www.aviva.com/newsroom/news-releases/2014/04/uk-first-time-parents-spend-492-million-preparing-for-baby-17298/

NICE guideline 'Postnatal care up to 8 weeks after birth', 2006. [ONLINE] available from www.nice.org.uk/guidance/cg37

Ou, H. *The first forty days, the essential art of nourishing the new mother,* Stewart, Tabori and Chang, 2016.

Packham, A. 'More Than 90% Of Mums Feel Lonely After Having Children And Many Don't Confide In Their Partner', 2017. [ONLINE] available from www.huffingtonpost.co.uk/entry/mums-feel-lonely-after-birth_uk_58bec088e4b09ab537d6bdf9

Placksin, S. *Mothering the new mother,* William Morrow, 1998.

Plett, H. 'What it means to "hold space" for people, plus eight tips on how to do it well', 2015[ONLINE] available from heatherplett.com/2015/03/hold-space/

Raven, JH, Chin, Q, Tolhurst, RJ and Garner P, 'Traditional beliefs and practices in the postpartum period in Fujian Province, China: a qualitative study', *BMC Pregnancy Childbirth,* 2007.

Rust, A. 'What do new mothers do all day?' [ONLINE] available from www.mother.ly/life/what-do-new-mothers-do-all-day, (no date).

Salmon, W. *The Works of Aristotle, The Famous Philosopher, in four parts*, London, 1791.

Scotland, M. *Why Postnatal Depression Matters,* Pinter & Martin, 2015.

Serralach, O. *The Postnatal Depletion Cure: A Complete Guide to*

Rebuilding Your Health and Reclaiming Your Energy for Mothers of Newborns, Toddlers and Young Children, Sphere, 2018.

Small, M. *Our babies, ourselves, how biology and culture shape the way we parent,* Anchor Books, 1998.

Smith, D. 'Shocking extent of loneliness faced by young mothers revealed', 2018. [ONLINE] available from www.co-operative.coop/media/news-releases/shocking-extent-of-loneliness-faced-by-young-mothers-revealed

Stadlen, N. *What Mothers Do especially when it looks like nothing,* Piatkus, 2004.

Stockton, A. *Gentle birth companions, doulas serving humanity,* McCubbington Press, 2010

Taylor E. *Becoming us, 8 steps to grow families that thrive,* Three Turtles Press, 2011.

Uvnas-Moberg, K. *The Hormone of Closeness,* Pinter & Martin, 2013.

Walne, E. 'The rise of the "monthly nurse"', 2011 [ONLINE] available from elizabethwalne.co.uk/blog/2011/2/22/the-rise-of-the-monthly-nurse.html

Williams, V. *Celebrating Life Customs around the World: From Baby Showers to Funerals,* ABC-CLIO, 2016.

Xu, Q., Séguin, L., Lise Goulet, L. 'Effet bénéfique d'un arrêt du travail avant l'accouchement', *Medicine* 2002

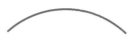

Index

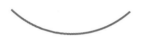

Series editor: Susan Last

pinterandmartin.com